The Vocal Instrument

The Vocal Instrument

SHARON L. RADIONOFF, Ph.D.

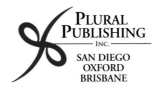

PLURAL
PUBLISHING
INC.
SAN DIEGO
OXFORD
BRISBANE

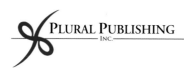

5521 Ruffin Road
San Diego, CA 92123

e-mail: info@pluralpublishing.com
Web site: http://www.pluralpublishing.com

49 Bath Street
Abingdon, Oxfordshire OX14 1EA
United Kingdom

Typeset in 11/13 Garamond by Flanagan's Publishing Services, Inc.
Printed in the Hong Kong by Paramount Printing

Library of Congress Cataloging-in-Publication Data:

Radionoff, Sharon L.
  The vocal instrument / Sharon L. Radionoff.
      p. cm.
   ISBN-13: 978-1-59756-163-1 (alk. paper)
   ISBN-10: 1-59756-163-0 (alk. paper)
   1. Voice—Care and hygiene. 2. Voice culture. 3. Voice disorders. 4. Singing—
Instruction and study. I. Title.
   MT821.R26 2008
   783—dc22
                                                                    2007048664

Contents

Foreword

*P*hysicians commonly see professional voice users who are passionate about their careers but their voices have broken down, jeopardizing job performance, and dream fulfillment. Tragically, many voice professionals have received little or no training about the human voice. They do not understand how it works, its fragility, its potential maladies, or how to maintain healthy and effective verbal communication. Although learning how to optimize the ability to communicate should be a requirement for all voice users, not only is this information scarce or absent in most education or training programs, but it is also hard to find in the literature even for those who recognize the need to learn more about their voices.

In *The Vocal Instrument*, Dr. Sharon Radionoff has provided a practical, well-grounded, and easily accessible resource. She has combined her experience as a singer, teacher, conductor (vocal and instrumental), and experienced medical singing voice specialist, to synthesize the key vocal problems encountered commonly by performers, voice pedagogues, conductors, and music educators. She has provided practical information on basic anatomy and physiology, identified factors that predispose to vocal failure and injury, and included practical guidelines and solutions to minimize risks, and optimize vocal health.

This book will be especially valuable for voice professionals who are at an exceptionally high risk for voice abuse and injury. The information is applicable to a wide array of voice dependent professionals in all fields, at all levels. It should be a valuable addition to the library of anyone who steps into a classroom or in front of an audience.

Robert T. Sataloff, M.D., D.M.A., F.A.C.S.
Professor and Chairman
Department of Otolaryngology–Head and Neck Surgery
Associate Dean for Clinical Academic Specialties
Drexel University College of Medicine

Introduction

Within the body lie all the elements (anatomy, physiology, and body/mind/spirit connection) that are needed to produce sound. Anatomy is our structure or what we are made of, whereas physiology is the function, or how we use our anatomy. Every instrument has a frame. The unique thing about the human vocal instrument is that the body skeleton is the frame. Because of this, singers must pay close attention to the way their "frame" is used. Inefficient alignment of body positioning can interfere with your "systems balance."

To create a dependable technique, there must be a balance of three main systems. These include balancing of the power source (respiratory system), the pitch source (phonatory system = vocal folds), and the quality shaper or resonator (supraglottic vocal tract = space above the vocal folds). When this balance does not exist, the singer will create compensations in order to try to achieve a desired sound. The singer does this because he hears something with his ears (his outside observers) which he does not like and controls to "fix" the sound.

There are certain areas where manipulations and problems frequently occur. The positioning of the postural elements will affect breath flow, breath support, resonance, and voice quality. Misalignment of the "frame" of your instrument will cause a chain of compensations to occur in your "systems balance." This can cause minor vocal difficulties that may eventually lead to significant pathologies.

The purpose of this book is to help the voice professional understand his or her instrument and know how to take care of it. The first half of this book answers the following questions: What is my instrument and how is it put together? How do I play it? and How do I take care of it? The second half of this book defines common problems and discusses how to fix them based on the specialization of the voice professional.

Preface

In 1965, a little boy wrote an essay that was published in the West Virginia Hospital News. The essay was on "Anatomy" or on "What Makes Up a Person" and here is what he said:

> Your head is kind of round and hard and your brains are in it and your hair is on it. Your face is the front of your head where you eat and make faces. Your neck is what keeps your head out of your collar. It's hard to keep clean. Your shoulders are sort of shelves where you hook your suspenders on them. Your stummick is something that if you don't eat often enough it hurts, and spinach don't help it none. Your spine is a long bone in your back that is always behind you no matter how quick you turn around. Your arms you got to have to pitch with and so you can reach the butter. Your fingers stick out of your hands so you can throw a curve and add up arithmetic. Your legs are what you run on, and your toes are what always get stubbed. And that's all there is of you except what's inside and I never saw it.

You probably had a little chuckle reading this story. Although it is written in the simplistic language of a child, it drives home a point to think about. What are the nuts and bolts of anatomy? What do we need to know about what comprises the vocal instrument? How is it put together? How do we play it and how do we keep it healthy? Some excellent books have been written about the voice but they demand a certain level of knowledge in order to gain insight from the writings. My desire is that this book will be a practical resource and spur the reader on to want to know more about the field of arts medicine and the voice.

Acknowledgments

I would like to thank the following people for their support and involvement in making this book possible:

Editorial Assistance—Leonard Radionoff, Jackie Gartner-Schmidt, Erin Lee, Ron Scherer, Kathy Knox, and Dell Mara Lovell

Contributions of thoughts and advice—Lee Poquette, John Gearhart, Steve Newberry, Cindy Cruise Ratcliff, John Kilgore, Doug Beiden, Scott Turnbull, Brian Philbin, Corey Trahan, Kirstina Driskill, Dan Vincent, and Jan Lewin.

Figures and pictures—Robert O'Brien (Blue Tree Publishing), C. Richard Stasney, Margarita Rodriguez, Lauren Bigelow (Texas Voice Center), Erin Lee (Sound Singing Institute), and Leonard Radionoff. St. Luke's United Methodist Church, West University Baptist Church, St. John the Divine Episcopal Church, Lakewood Church, House of Refuge Christian Church, and Alief Church of Christ.

To all of my clients, colleagues and friends who were willing pictorial participants: Crisi Carter, Melina Gonzalez, Dr. Robert T. Sataloff, Brenda Beiden, Becky Simon, Doug Beiden, Stacey Weber, Debbie Fancher, Lee Poquette, Aaron Rodriguez, John Kilgore, Brian Philbin, Robert Simpson, Corey Trahan, Katherine Ciesinski, John Gremillion, Kitty Karn, Tracy Rhodus Satterfield, April Rapier, Doyle Bramhall (Barbara Logan too), Diane Landry, Rosalyn Brunswick-McDuffie, Walter Suhr, Kristina Driskill, and Todd Waite. Thank you also to all the photographers who assisted in this process.

To my mentor, colleague and friend Dr. Robert T. Sataloff, who gave me the opportunity to become involved in the specialized field of Professional Voice Care and continues to mentor and support me.

This book is dedicated to my parents, Leonard and Linda Radionoff, with overflowing, deep, heartfelt gratitude for their never ending love, support, and constant encouragement. Thank you for always having a spot open at "Chez Radionoff" and thank you dad for being my chief editor!

It is your love and support that made this book possible.

Chapter 1

What Is My Instrument and How Is It Put Together?

*W*here does the impulse for sound begin? In the larynx? No! In the brain (Figure 1-1). This fact alone should go a long way to help a singer understand that he/she does not have to "work hard at the larynx" (throat area) to make sound better. In fact, the more that one manipulates and tries to control the sound (often meaning squeezing with neck muscles) the less one's vocal system is able to achieve freedom and flexibility of sound.[1] The creation of basic sound incorporates three main systems; the respiratory system (power source), the phonatory system (pitch source), and the supraglottic vocal tract or resonance tract (quality shaper).[2] Along with this is also the articulatory system. This chapter examines (1) the instrument frame, (2) three main systems of sound production, (3) articulation, and (4) the body/mind/spirit connection.

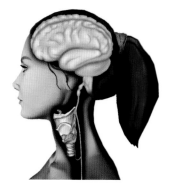

Figure 1-1. Sagittal (*side*) view of the brain, nerves, and laryngeal skeleton.

Body

Instrument Frame

Every musical instrument has a frame and the voice is no different. The skeletal frame of the body is the frame of the vocal instrument (Figures 1–2A–C).[2] Therefore, body alignment (what is often referred to as posture), movement, dance, and choreography all have the potential to affect vocal sound. Body alignment and efficiency are not about a static, rigid, still posture. It is about answering questions like: where is my center of gravity as I move through various positions in space, and what possibilities exist? There are excellent methods one can study in regard to body work and sound such as Feldenkrais, Alexander technique, and the Linklater technique. Yoga is another excellent pursuit which helps stretch and open up the body for more elasticity and efficiency for pre-eminent body response.

Because the physical body is the instrument, it is about training the body (the systems necessary) to respond in order to be able to express what one wants to express. How does one do this? By setting

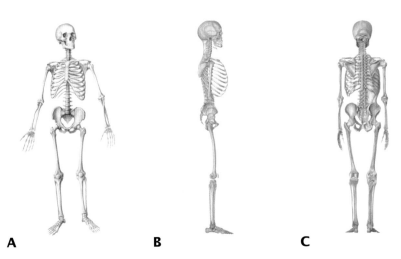

A   **B**   **C**

Figure 1–2. **A.** Front view of the skeleton (frame of the vocal instrument). **B.** Side view of the skeleton (frame of the vocal instrument). **C.** Back view of the skeleton (frame of the vocal instrument).

up the environment with exercises that bring about the necessary brain/body response so that the body can respond how one wants it to respond without excessive energy or manipulative pushing, pulling, yanking, or shoving.

Experimentation and Awareness

Alignment and efficiency of body energy may be evaluated from standing, sitting, and movement positions. In order to have efficient use of body energy and movement, one needs to experiment with extremes of positions to find his/her personal midpoint, much as a pendulum swings from side to side but always passes through a midpoint. It is essential to be aware of how one is put together (anatomy/structure) and what one is doing (physiology/function) to understand what is efficient. If there is need for any change then awareness is critical. Without awareness no change can occur. There may be a difference between habitual alignment (how one has trained the body) and actual/natural/efficient alignment. Furthermore, there will be alignment differences for every person based on physical issues such as scoliosis and so forth. Also, there will be other issues to consider if one is wheelchair bound or has had surgery. Efficient function of the instrument frame will allow for the most elasticity and efficiency for the respiratory system (the power source of sound). The first body position to be examined in regard to efficiency is standing.

Standing Alignment (basic stance):

- Feet may be somewhere between a few inches apart and shoulder width apart
- Find the center of gravity of your body weight.
  - Experiment with body weight. Move the body weight front and back to find the center of gravity. Notice that the body weight too far forward toward the toes makes one feel off balance. Notice that body weight too far back on the heels locks the knees.
- Knees should be flexible and relaxed, not rigid and tense
  - Hips should be aligned such that the lower back is not excessively arched as seen in Figure 1–3A. This overarching will not allow the abdominal muscles to be used efficiently for exhalation.

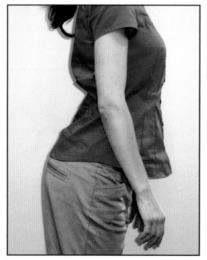 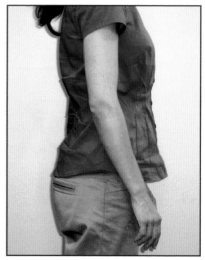

A   **B**

***Figure 1-3.* A.** Overextension of hip position. **B.** Midpoint hip position (natural alignment).

- o Put your hands on your hips. Rotate and rock the pelvis/hips front and back to find your midpoint (Figure 1-3B). While you are doing this be sure to keep your upper torso still.
- ■ Shoulders should not be too far forward (Figure 1-4A) or pulled back too far in a military stance (Figure 1-4B).
- ■ Upper torso/sternum should not be caved in (Figure 1-4A) or pulled back (Figure 1-4B).
  - o A useful way to find a good shoulder/upper torso position (Figure 1-4C) is to put your arms straight up above your head with your palms together. Slowly bring your arms down at your sides (arms still straight not bent at the elbows) with you palms facing up to the sky. When your arms get to about the 4 o' clock position stop, rotate your palms in and let your arms fall down to your body.
- ■ Head/neck position. It is difficult to feel and find an efficient head/neck position by oneself. The Alexander technique is excellent for this alignment.
  - o Try an experiment. Let you head fall back like you have fallen asleep. Put the palm of one hand at the nape of your

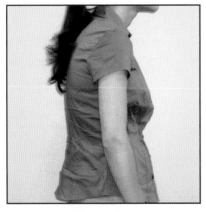

A

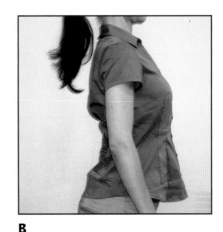

B

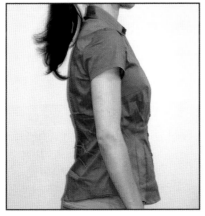

C

Figure 1–4. **A.** Shoulders too far forward and upper torso/sternum caved in. **B.** Shoulders pulled too far back and upper torso/sternum pulled high and back. **C.** Midpoint shoulder and upper torso/sternum position (natural alignment).

neck. Try elevating the back of your head so that it rests over your spine. Try not to push the head forward or to press your chin back. Follow the steps below in regard to position and angle of the ears.

- o Protrusion—it is often very common to find jutting or sticking out of the neck with the head so far forward that the ears are no longer over the shoulders (Figure 1-5). A general rule of thumb for head/neck position is that the ears are over the shoulders and the neck is in line with the torso.
- o Elevation—can happen when looking up at someone taller or sitting looking up at a screen that is too close (Figure 1-6).

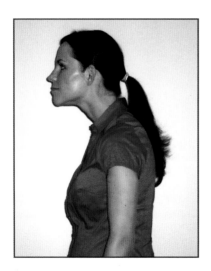

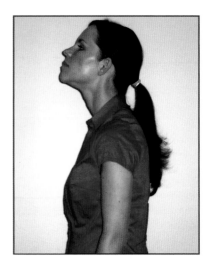

Figure 1–5. Head and neck protrusion.

Figure 1–6. Head and neck elevation.

Elevating the head may also go along with protrusion (Figure 1-7). You can check the angle of the ears to see if they are straight over the shoulders or if they angle with the earlobe pointing forward. Remember: the rule of thumb is that the ears are straight over the shoulders.

o Tucking—often in the attempt to find an efficient head/neck position, the chin is tucked back and down (Figure 1-8). This chin position is most likely not beneficial because there will be tension and pressure of the extrinsic muscles of the larynx (neck muscles) and potentially stop flexibility of the voice.

o Compression—it is very common for the head and back of the neck to be compressed down (Figure 1-9). Think about what happens to your head/neck position when you slouch or when you get tired. This position adds pressure at the neck/larynx. Any unnecessary pressure/tension has potentially unhealthy ramifications down the road (compare Figure 1-10, normal alignment).

■ Jaw position

o Mandibular restriction—it is necessary to evaluate if there is any medical or functional restriction of the jaw since the

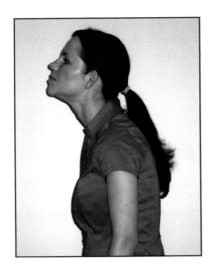

Figure 1-7. Head and neck combination of protrusion and elevation.

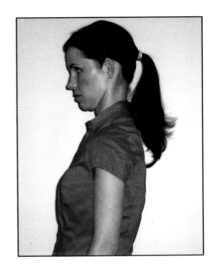

Figure 1-8. Chin tucking.

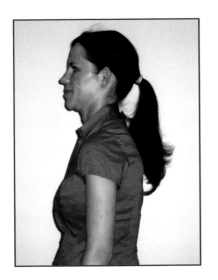

Figure 1-9. Neck compression.

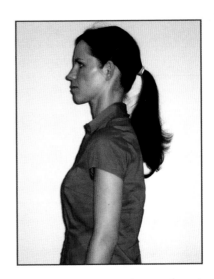

Figure 1-10. Midpoint head and neck natural alignment.

jaw position is directly related to sound quality. TMD (temporal mandibular dysfunction) or TMJ (Temporal mandibular joint dysfunction) is a jaw issue that can greatly affect the physiology and psychology of a singer. This is a condition where the jaw pops and clicks and there can be referred ear/back/neck pain. It is often said to be primarily stress related but also may be, in fact, related to bite issues with the upper and lower teeth.

o Jaw jutting—again this can be a medical condition of lower jaw protrusion or it can be a habitual/functional issue. As above, this can affect the singer and articulatory issues may occur.

Sitting Alignment: The position of the lower back when sitting is an important issue. Often one has been told to "sit up straight." The problem is that this command is translated into an inefficient position of overarching the lower back which will affect the ability of the abdominal muscles to work maximally for exhalation.

■ Try an experiment:
  o Sit on the edge of a chair and hyperarch the lower back and overlift the chest. Notice how uncomfortable and stiff this feels (Figure 1–11A).
  o Next, let the hips roll back and experience how the body weight sinks down into the chair so that the lower back relaxes its hyperextension (Figure 1–11B). Be aware that there are two separate movements possible: a waist-up half of body movement that bends forward and back, and a hip movement that flexes and releases. It may feel like the body has to totally collapse when the hips rock back and the body weight sinks into the chair (Figure 1–11C). This is not true as the upper half of the torso, from the waist up, can be nicely aligned and efficient while still being relaxed.[3]

A cautionary note needs to be inserted when examining alignment: Movement is allowed and necessary. Sometimes in the effort to find alignment we create tension and rigidity by trying to create a perfect, stationary alignment. Remember that the objective is not to be a statue or sculpture, but to be flexible, elastic, and responsive. It is highly beneficial to practice airflow and phonation exercises in many positions such as the multitasking exercises found in Chapter 2. When

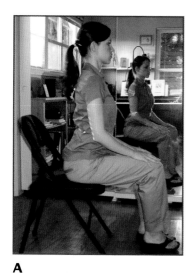

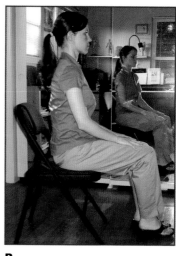

A

B

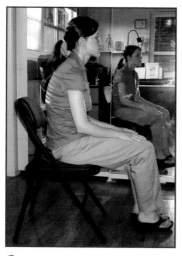

C

Figure 1–11. **A.** Overextension of the lower back while sitting. **B.** Relaxed natural low back alignment while sitting. **C.** Collapse of upper torso while sitting.

singers perform they usually move and do not stay still. Freedom of movement and expression for the performer is critical. Discussion of detailed movement issues is beyond the scope of this chapter because they demand visual observation as a number of variables are involved.

Respiration

Basic Anatomy and Physiology

The respiratory system is the power source of sound and is composed of two processes: inhalation and exhalation. Inhalation (air coming in) is always an active process. This is because the diaphragm (a double dome-shaped structure of muscle and tendon) must contract in order for breath to come into the lungs. There is much misconception about the respiratory system and, in particular, the diaphragm. Many people put their hands on their abdomen (stomach) and say "breathe from your diaphragm."[4] Let us first clear up myth #1—location of the diaphragm. The diaphragm is not located where the hands are on the abdomen as discussed above. In fact, if the skin were taken away from the abdomen you would not see the diaphragm but what we collectively call the abdominal muscles. The diaphragm is like a double dome or bowl turned upside down and tipped up slightly in the front. It connects to the breastbone or sternum in the front, to the ribs all the way around the body, and to the spine in the back. The dome is also lower on the side where the heart is located to make room for the heart. It separates the chest (thorax) from the stomach (abdomen/viscera) (Figures 1–12A and 1–12B, and 1–13).[4]

Myth #2—telling people to "breathe from the diaphragm" needs clarification. This is actually a silly statement because if the diaphragm were to stop working we would die. It is an involuntary muscle and must work in order for breath to come into the body. When the body needs breath, the brain fires information to the respiratory system and the double-dome shaped structure called the diaphragm contracts or flattens. This in turn pulls open the ribs which pulls open the lungs. This action of the lungs creates a partial vacuum and sucks air into the lungs. This takes care of what happens above the diaphragm (thorax or chest area) but what happens below the diaphragm?

When the diaphragm contracts and pushes against the innards (viscera-stomach/intestines/etc.) they need to move. Thus, the stomach expands and "pooches" out. If the stomach is held tight and rigid, airflow will still be able to move in and out but there will not be maximum benefit or efficient use of the respiratory system for the power source (breath support/breath control) of sound.

The process of exhalation (air going out) can be passive, active, or somewhere in between. An example of passive would be when a person is sitting watching TV and the diaphragm simply relaxes its

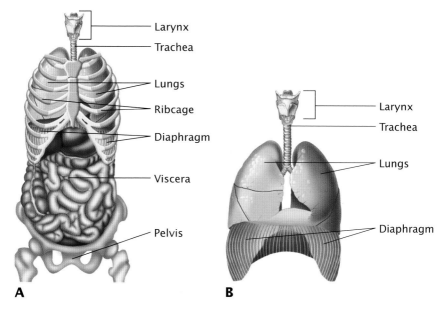

Figure 1-12. **A.** Front view of the torso including the lungs, ribcage, diaphragm, viscera, and pelvis. **B.** Front view of the torso including the lungs and diaphragm.

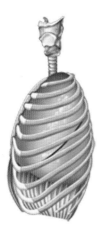

Figure 1-13. Side view inhalation.

contraction and pushes air out of the lungs. An example of active would be like yelling "Hey" in a panic situation. This activity uses forceful contraction of the abdominal muscles for active exhalation. For singing, the goal is to train a steady, managed airflow which some people call breath control/support.

The primary muscles of exhalation are collectively called the abdominal muscles (Figure 1–14). They include the rectus abdominus, transversus abdominus, and internal and external obliques.[5] There are also rib muscles; the internal and external intercostals, as well as back muscles. The respiratory system works like a bellows. Air in = tummy pooches out, air out = tummy comes back in (Figure 1–15). If you don't believe it or can't feel the stomach pooch out when air comes in and then the space goes away when breath leaves, go to the exercises in Chapter 2. Singing different types of music and/or phrases require different amounts of breath. It is highly beneficial for the singer to train the ability to access minimum and maximum amounts of managed airflow. The objective is to train managed airflow to achieve consistency of phonation. After consistency of steady phonation is achieved one can move to the more athletic endeavors of musicality (i.e., crescendo/diminuendo—loud/soft).

Phonation

The phonatory system is the pitch source of our instrument. Before examining the structure of the larynx in more detail, let's take a brief peak at an internal view of the vocal folds (vocal cords). The vocal folds sit across the trachea horizontally. Figure 1–16A shows the loca-

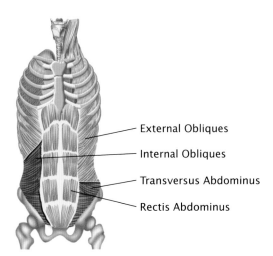

External Obliques

Internal Obliques

Transversus Abdominus

Rectis Abdominus

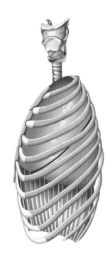

Figure 1–14. Front view of what are commonly called the abdominal muscles.

Figure 1–15. Side view exhalation.

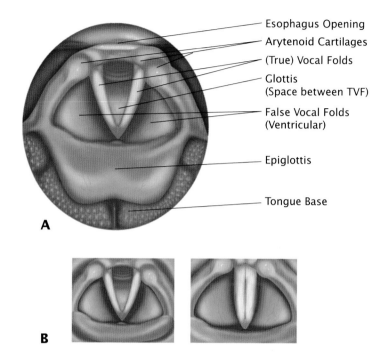

Figure 1-16. **A.** Internal view of the true vocal folds, false vocal folds (ventricular folds), arytenoid cartilages, epiglottis, and tongue base. **B.** Closer internal view of the true vocal folds, false vocal folds, and part of the epiglottis and arytenoid cartilages.

tion of the epiglottis and tongue base along with the opening to the esophagus. Figure 1-16B is a closer view of an open and closed view of the glottis (space between the vocal folds). It is important to remember when looking at pictures taken with an endoscope that the view is from above looking down the throat at the top surface of the vocal folds. The vocal folds may appear vertical on the screen but they are not. Remember: they sit across the trachea horizontally. Also, a camera flips the images; right is the left side of the vocal folds and the left side is the right vocal fold.

The Basic Anatomy of Sound

The structure of the larynx is composed of four basic anatomic components: Cartilaginous skeleton, intrinsic muscles, extrinsic muscles, and mucosa or soft lining.[6] These cartilages are made of hyaline and can ossify or harden. Ossification can begin in a person as early as puberty or not happen until one's middle sixties.[7]

First Component. The skeleton has three cartilages of primary importance: the thyroid cartilage, cricoid cartilage, and a pair of arytenoid cartilages. Other skeleton components include the epiglottis, hyoid bone, and corniculate cartilage (Figures 1–17, 1–18A and 1–18B, and 1–19).[6]

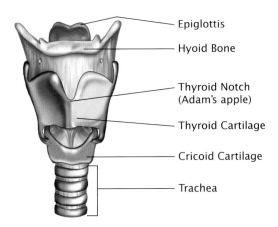

Epiglottis
Hyoid Bone
Thyroid Notch (Adam's apple)
Thyroid Cartilage
Cricoid Cartilage
Trachea

Figure 1–17. Front view of the laryngeal skeleton.

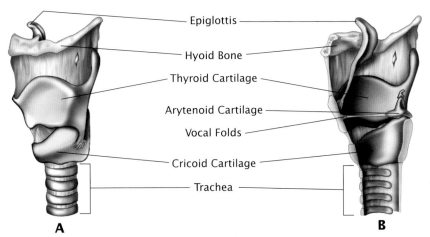

Epiglottis
Hyoid Bone
Thyroid Cartilage
Arytenoid Cartilage
Vocal Folds
Cricoid Cartilage
Trachea

A   **B**

Figure 1–18. **A.** Side view of the laryngeal skeleton. **B.** Side-cut side view of the laryngeal skeleton. It shows the epiglottis and vocal fold attachments.

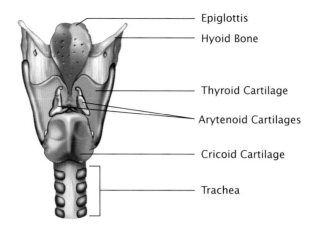

Figure 1-19. Back view of the laryngeal skeleton.

The names of the cartilages are actually very logical. The name thyroid is derived from the Greek word *thyri* that means shieldlike, but the combining form *thyro* denotes a relationship to the thyroid gland.[8] There is a notch at the front portion of the thyroid cartilage that is called the thyroid notch. This notch is more prominent in men than in women and we call this notch the Adam's apple (see Figures 1-17 and 1-18A and 1-18B).

The name of the cricoid cartilage is derived from the Greek word *krikos* that means ring plus *eidos* which means form = *ringlike form*. The structure was actually compared to the ring used by Turkish archers (see Figures 1-17, 1-18A, and 1-18B).[8]

The name for the paired arytenoid cartilages is derived from the Greek work *arytaina* which means "ladle" plus *eidos* which means "form" = *ladlelike form*.[8] The epiglottis is a leaflike cartilaginous structure. The prefix "*epi*" is a Greek work that means on or above and *glottis* refers to the space between the vocal folds. Therefore, the epiglottis is located on or above the space between the vocal folds (see Figure 1-19).

The name for the hyoid bone is derived from the Greek word *hyoeides*, which means U-shaped and was thus named because it is shaped like the Greek letter *upsilon* (see Figures 1-17 and 1-18A and 1-18B).[8]

Second Component. The intrinsic muscles, the second component, run between the cartilages. The names of these muscles are derived from the corresponding cartilages (e.g., cricoarytenoid = cricoid + arytenoid cartilages). The pair of intrinsic muscles that form the body of the vocal folds are the thyroarytenoid (TA), or vocalis, muscles. This pair extends from the arytenoid cartilage to a point inside the thyroid cartilage, just below the Adam's apple.[6]

Intrinsic muscles can change the position of the cartilages and pull them through a series of motions. This in turn alters the shape, position, and tension of the vocal folds. The intrinsic muscles can be categorized as either those that are *ab*ducting (pulling apart) or those that are *add*ucting (bringing together) the vocal folds.[6]

The principal muscle of *ab*duction is the posterior cricoarytenoid (PCA). As we look at Figure 1–20 we can see that this muscle is located at the back (posterior) of the laryngeal skeleton and connects from the cricoid to the arytenoid cartilages.[6]

The principle muscles of *add*uction are thought to be the lateral cricoarytenoid (LCA) and interarytenoid (IA).[8] Other muscles of *add*uction include the thyroarytenoid (TA) and cricothyroid (CT). As we look at Figure 1–21 we can see where the TA muscle is located. Remember that this muscle makes up the body of the vocal folds. It connects at the anterior (front) inside portion of the thyroid cartilage just below the thyroid notch (Adam's apple) and to the arytenoid cartilages at the posterior (back) position of the laryngeal skeleton.[6]

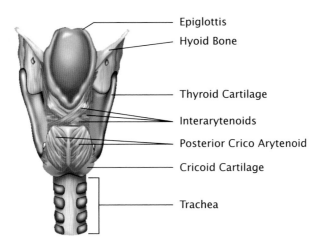

Epiglottis
Hyoid Bone

Thyroid Cartilage

Interarytenoids

Posterior Crico Arytenoid

Cricoid Cartilage

Trachea

Figure 1–20. Principal muscle of abduction— posterior cricoarytenoid (PCA). Principal muscles of adduction include the interanytenoid (IA).

The lateral cricoarytenoid connects from the cricoid across (hence lateral) to the opposite arytenoid cartilage. The interarytenoid muscle consists of both transverse and oblique fibers. The interarytenoid muscle is seen in Figure 1–20.[6]

The cricothyroid connects from the cricoid to the thyroid as seen in Figures 1–22A and B. This muscle, the CT, is the principle muscle for stretching or longitudinal tension. What does this mean in terms of function? It means that this muscle must become more activated in order for us to be able to phonate higher pitches.

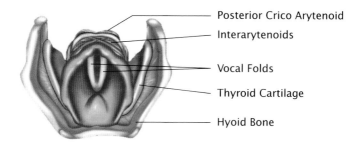

Figure 1–21. Principal muscles of adduction include the thyroarytenoid (TA). This muscle also comprises the body of the vocal folds.

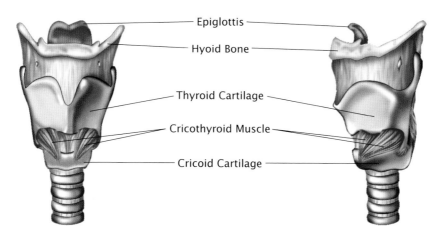

Figure 1–22. Principal muscles of adduction include cricothyroid (CT). This is also the principle muscle for stretching or longitudinal tension. **A.** Front view, **B.** Side view.

All of the muscles mentioned above must be innervated (told what to do) by something in order to function. That means information must move from the brain through nerves to these muscles. The recurrent and superior laryngeal nerves, branches of the vagus cranial nerve, control the intrinsic muscles in the larynx (Figure 1-23). The main responsibility of the superior laryngeal nerve is to innervate the CT muscle and the recurrent laryngeal nerve innervates the rest of the intrinsic muscles (TA or vocalis, PCA, LCA, and IA).[6]

Third Component. The third component of the larynx is the extrinsic muscles. These muscles are called this because they refer to the muscles that are external or outside the laryngeal skeleton. These muscles connect the cartilages to other throat structures. They are commonly referred to as the strap muscles of the neck (Figure 1-24). They raise and lower the entire laryngeal skeleton and are divided into

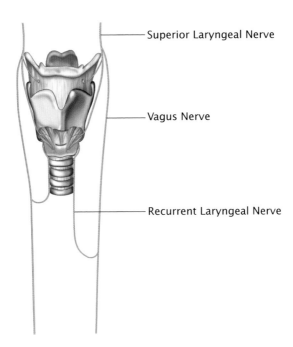

Superior Laryngeal Nerve

Vagus Nerve

Recurrent Laryngeal Nerve

Figure 1-23. The superior and recurrent laryngeal nerves, branches of the 10th cranial nerve (vagus nerve), which innervate the intrinsic muscles of the larynx.

two categories: Those that are below the hyoid bone (see Figures 1-17 and 1-18 for hyoid bone location) and those that are above the hyoid bone. Those below the hyoid bone are called infrahyoid muscles (because they connect from the hyoid bone down or one could say they are "inside") and those above the hyoid bone are called suprahyoid muscles (because they connect from the hyoid bone and up or one could say they are "above"). The infrahyoid muscles include the thyrohyoid, sternothyroid, sternohyoid and omohyoid. The suprahyoid muscles include the digastric, mylohyoid, geniohyoid, and stylohyoid (Figures 1-25 and 1-26). [6,7]

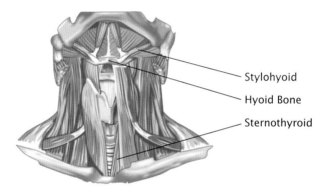

Stylohyoid

Hyoid Bone

Sternothyroid

Figure 1-24. Extrinsic laryngeal muscles commonly referred to as the strap muscles of the neck.

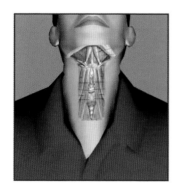

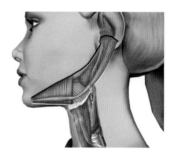

Figure 1-25. Front view of the suprahyoid and infrahyoid extrinsic laryngeal muscles.

Figure 1-26. Side view of the suprahyoid and infrahyoid extrinsic laryngeal muscles.

Fourth Component. The final component of the larynx is the mucosa or smooth lubricated surface. The tissues lining the larynx are much more complex than was originally understood. In 1975, physician Minoru Hirano made important discoveries that revolutionized the understanding and treatment of the vocal folds. Identification of five distinct layers in the structure of the vocal fold are as follows: a thin lubricated epithelium, three layers of tissue called the lamina propria (superficial, intermediate, and deep layers), and the deep muscle layer which is composed of the thyroarytenoid muscle (TA).[9,10] In practical terms, these five layers can be discussed as three basic layers including a (1) cover, (2) transition layer, and (3) body. The cover is composed of the epithelium and superficial lamina propria, the transition layer is composed of the intermediate and deep lamina propria layers, whereas the body is composed of the thyroarytenoid or vocalis muscle (Figure 1-27).[10]

The Basic Physiology of Sound

Now that the anatomy of sound has been examined, it is worthwhile to track where sound begins and how it travels. The impulse for making sound begins in the cerebral cortex of the brain and then information is sent through the 10th cranial nerve to the appropriate laryngeal muscles.[10] During phonation, the ear (Figure 1-28) picks up sound produced by the vocal system and regulates the shaping of the vocal

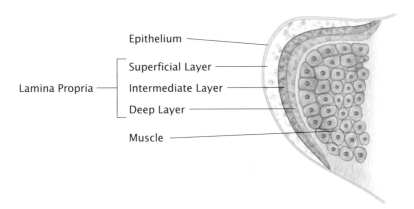

Figure 1-27. A frontal section of the human vocal fold through the middle of the membranous portion.

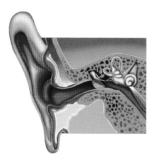

Figure 1–28. Side-cut view of the ear.

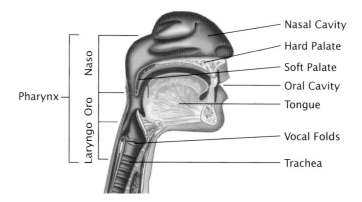

Figure 1–29. Side-cut view of the supraglottic vocal tract (SVT).

tract (Figure 1–29) to "sculpt" the sound. This feedback system is used by the brain to try to match the *actual* sound of the voice with the sound *intended* by the communication centers of the brain that generate the voice.[11] The creation of basic sound incorporates three main systems; the respiratory system (power source), the phonatory system (pitch source), and the supraglottic vocal tract or resonance tract (quality shaper). Along with this is the articulatory system. Chart 1–1 illustrates the flow of the physiology of sound.[12]

Theory of Phonation. Understanding voice production is based on the myoelastic-aerodynamic theory of phonation. This incorporates both the properties of the vocal folds (mass, elasticity, damping) and

Physiology

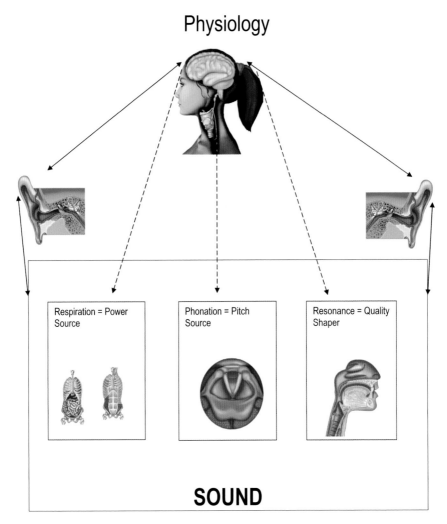

Respiration = Power Source

Phonation = Pitch Source

Resonance = Quality Shaper

SOUND

Chart 1–1

aerodynamic pressures and flows (air pressures acting on the vocal folds and airflow through the glottis).[13-15] Simply stated, when the vocal folds are close to each other, sufficient lung pressure provides enough air pressure to push the two vocal folds away from each other slightly. The vocal folds then recoil back toward each other due to their elasticity along with airflow properties. Figure 1–30A shows a side-cut view (coronal view) of the vocal folds and surrounding anat-

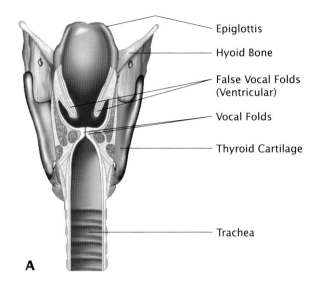

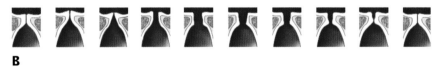

Figure 1–30. **A.** Side-cut view of the larynx. **B.** Vibratory cycle of the vocal folds.

omy. Figure 1–30B shows a side-cut view of the vocal fold vibratory cycle. For a more complete discussion of the myoelastic-aerodynamic theory of phonation, refer to Scherer[14] and Titze.[15,16]

Music and the Brain

The idea of sound beginning in the cerebral cortex has been discussed above but where does the singer (musician) process music? Brain function, as it relates to music has often been relegated to activity in the right hemisphere of the brain. However, Pribram[17] cited that not only are different aspects of music processed in both hemispheres, but that semantic reference (the meaning of signs—what they refer to), and pragmatic meaning (how signs relate to the user) are processed separately. Furthermore, Wilson[18] proposed a theory in which he stated that all of us have a biologic guarantee of musicianship. Recent findings indicate that music does have a biological basis and that the brain has a functional organization for music. Furthermore, it seems that many brain regions play a part in specific aspects of music processing. It also appears that musicians have hyperdevelopment of some brain structures.[19]

Resonance

Every instrument has a resonating body (cavity or tube) which is the quality shaper for sound or *timbre* (pronounced tamber) for that particular instrument. It is the *timbre* that makes each instrument unique and recognizable. The interesting aspect for a singer/voice user is that the resonating cavity is within the head and has many variables that can change. The resonator of the vocal instrument is called the supraglottic vocal tract (SVT). Supra means above, glottis refers to the space between the vocal folds, vocal means voice, and tract means area. Therefore, the SVT refers to the space from just above the vocal folds all the way out to the lips. The singer's resonator, the supraglottic vocal tract, is composed of the supraglottic larynx, tongue, lips, palate, pharynx, and nasal cavity.[6] It is capable of being altered in shape by the following: (1) jaw position may be changed, (2) tongue position may be altered (has complex connections to the larynx, pharynx, and soft palate),[7] (3) the soft palate may be changed, (4) the lips may be altered, (5) the mouth opening may be changed, and (6) the vertical height of the larynx position may be altered (see Figure 1-29).

Pharynx

The pharynx (back wall of the throat—BWT) has three parts; nasopharynx (BWT behind the nose), oropharynx (BWT behind the mouth), and the laryngopharynx (BWT near the larynx). There are major landmarks to which the pharynx (BWT) is attached. Important attachments include (1) the hard palate, (2) hyoid bone, (3) thyroid cartilage, and (4) cricoid cartilage. There are three important groups of paired muscles that contribute to the shape of the pharynx: the pharyngeal constrictors, slender longitudinal muscles, and the muscles of the soft palate. The pharyngeal constrictors lessen the width of the pharynx when contracted. The relatively slender longitudinal muscles shorten the length of the pharynx. The soft palate may be elevated by contracting levator veli palatini muscles and may be pulled horizontally when the tensor veli palatini muscles are activated.[7]

Singers are sometimes told that they do not have resonance—this is not a true statement as all living humans have a head! It is more accurate to define what kind of resonance is occurring. Examples of resonance may include hypernasality, hyponasality, laryngeal resonance, and head voice resonance or called resonant voice. Hyper—refers to too much—that the velopharyngeal port (opening between nose and throat) is too open, and hypo—refers to absence—that the velopharyngeal port is not open enough. Laryngeal resonance is a term used by some speech-language pathologists (SLP) to define sound that is resonating back in the throat. Head voice resonance, or resonant voice, is another speech-language pathology term that defines sound as resonating frontally—some voice teachers call this resonating in the "mask."

Basic Acoustics of the Vocal Tract

The function of vibratory action of the vocal folds is basically opposite to that of a stringed instrument. When a guitar string is plucked, the plucking action excites and vibrates the air. However, with the vocal folds, it is the air (lung pressure + Bernoulli pressure), innervation from the two branches (superior and recurrent laryngeal nerves) of the 10th (vagus) cranial nerve and the elasticity of the vocal folds that allows vibratory action to occur. The vocal folds are pushed apart and are sucked back together. Each separation and collision creates a puff of air in the vocal tract. The number of times per second that the vocal folds separate and collide determines the number of air puffs that escape; or rather the number of occurrences of frequency. The frequency of the vocal fold opening and closing is perceived as pitch and is measured in hertz (i.e., Middle C = 262 Hz) (Figures 1–31 and 1–32).[6]

The sound at the vocal fold level, or glottal wave source, is equal to a buzz; however, it contains a fundamental frequency with a complete set of harmonic partials or overtones. The sound then passes from the larynx through the supraglottic vocal tract. The shape of the SVT is determined by vowel and consonant production and the desired timbre or sound quality. The harmonics which become strengthened as they pass through the resonator are called **formant frequencies**.[20]

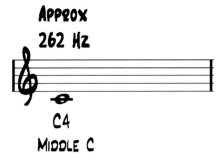

APPROX
262 Hz

C4
MIDDLE C

Figure 1–31. Middle C (C4 acoustic number designation).

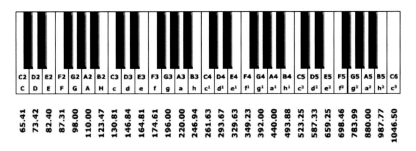

Figure 1–32. Keyboard showing corresponding Hertz with acoustic and musical pitch number designations.

These pitch areas, or formants are often discussed in terms of the peak of the area rather than the entire pitch area. There are primarily four or five formants of interest. The two lowest formants determine most of the vowel color whereas the third, fourth, and fifth formants are of greater significance to voice timbre. It is possible to see an acoustical voice print of changes that occur within the vocal tract when articulation changes. In Figure 1–33 one can see how a change in vowel formation changes the strengths of formants 1 and 2. These changes are created mainly by tongue position alteration and to some extent the lips (for the /u/ and /o/ vowels). There is little or no movement of the lower jaw.[20]

When formants 3 to 5 cluster together a unique phenomenon occurs. The "Singer's Formant or Speaker's Ring" is the "ring" or "ping" that allow a voice to be heard over an orchestra without a microphone. The singer's formant ranges from 2400 to 3200 Hz depending

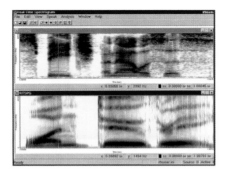

Figure 1-33. Spectrogram.

on the voice category. The research of resonance in regard to singing has primarily been aimed toward western classical singing. However, other genres/styles of singing within the United States and other countries are now beginning to be researched.

Vocal Tract/Sound Quality/Face Shape

Face shape—from the side of the face, the shape from cheek to jaw to lips is essentially an isosceles triangle (Figure 1-34) (or in three dimensions an inverted megaphone or pyramid) (Figure 1-35). A singer's job is to maximize what is natural. Once a singer knows the balance of one's instrument then one can discover how far from center point of the system's balance one can travel without losing balance.

Overwork for Lower Jaw Release. If overwork for lower jaw release occurs, then the back wall of the pharynx pulls down as does the soft palate. This in turn creates a dark sound which may also sound flat in pitch perception to the ears because the mid-upper harmonics have been dampened, even if the vocal folds are vibrating the correct number of times per second to create a given pitch (Figure 1-36).

Overwork for Upper "Lift." If overwork for upper lift (sometimes showing upper teeth excessively) occurs, then the back wall of the pharynx is pulled up, the soft palate is overlifted/raised, and sometimes the jaw is tensed and the vertical position of the larynx is either raised or rigid. This, in turn, creates an overly bright, edgy metalliclike sound and also sharp in pitch perception to the ears because the

Cheek

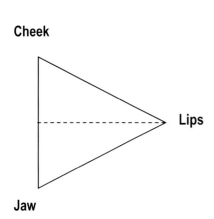

Lips

Jaw

Figure 1–34. Face shape from the side.

Cheek

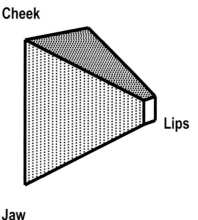

Lips

Jaw

Figure 1–35. Three-dimensional face shape from the side.

Cheek   Lips

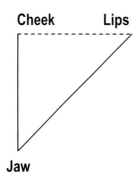

Jaw

Figure 1–36. Face shape changes from an isosceles triangle to a right-angle triangle.

mid-lower harmonics have been dampened, even if the vocal folds are vibrating the correct number of times per second to create a given pitch (Figure 1–37).

Vocal Quality

There are many sounds that one is capable of making. It is important to know what the central balance point of one's sound is before experimenting outside an efficient balance. This is beneficial for longevity of singing with freedom and minimized risk of vocal problems. Bunch

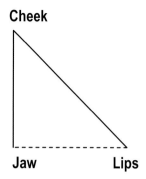

Cheek

Jaw   **Lips**

Figure 1–37. Face changes from isosceles triangle to another type of right-angle triangle.

describes four major components of a singer that can have a bearing on his/her vocal quality. These are (1) the physical structure of the head, neck, and vocal tract, (2) the co-ordination of the mechanism for singing, (3) the imagination of the singer, and (4) the levels of health and energy. Bunch further defines main factors that affect vocal quality. These factors include: (1) muscular overreaction (facial muscles, position and movement of the lower jaw, rigidity of the tongue, tension in the neck, tension in the chest), (2) emotional tension and (3) medical/physical issues.[7] Currently the most noninvasive and easiest way to examine vocal quality is through acoustic measurements. These are discussed in the third chapter of this book "How Do I Take Care of It?"

Articulation

Have you ever tried to clearly communicate after having had Novocain for a dental procedure? It is difficult to feel like you can talk (i.e., articulate clearly) when the tongue/lips feels like lead. What is articulation? Simply put, it is the ability to form words. It is the function of the articulatory system that allows for understandable communication. How this system is used determines the efficiency and clarity of what we do. For precise articulation we don't need to overdo, we just need to know what to do. During articulation there is a shifting or shaping of the resonance tract which sort of resembles a constantly morphing or changing "cartoon-like" trumpet.[21]

Mechanism

Members of the articulatory system are separated into two categories: fixed and movable structures. The fixed structures act as a foundation for the movable structures. The fixed structures include the teeth, aveolar ridge supporting the teeth (bony ridge behind the teeth), and the hard palate.

The movable structures are the lower jaw (mandible), lips, tongue, and soft palate.[7]

Although the jaw is often called an articulator, I believe it is clearer to state that it is part of the articulatory system but does not initiate articulation. It needs to be "free to flap in the breeze" but not act as an instigator. This is difficult because the muscles of the jaw are used primarily for clenching, biting, grinding, and chewing. In fact, the muscles controlling the lower jaw are the most powerful muscles in the head.[7] This poses a problem, because when singing, one is asking the muscles to release and not contract, which is the opposite of the earlier mentioned activities. Generally, whatever is the strongest and most used behavior of a muscle or muscle group is what we tend to gravitate toward first. Also, many singers overwork the jaw because they've been told things like: "chew your words," enunciate clearly, and that often translates into excessive work, not more precise work.

Vowels. Vowels are primarily shaped inside the vocal tract by the tongue and for the vowels */u/ and */o/, the lips must be round and oval, respectively. Singers who study voice are surprised to learn how little the mouth shape has to do with most vowels and they are also surprised that they don't have to create the vowel with an onset at the vocal folds; the vocal folds themselves have nothing to do with creating a vowel sound. Also a common misconception and misperception is that the lips must pull back into a smiling position in order for an accurate /i/ vowel. This is not necessary as only the tongue shape and position are needed for this vowel production.

Consonants. Consonants are organized by type/classification and anatomic area as well as the manner of shaping of the speech sounds below (see Figure 1–29).[8]

---

*International Phonetic Alphabet—see comparison chart for vowels in Chapter 2.

■ Class and Anatomic Area
  o Lips = labial/bilabial
  o Teeth = dental
  o Lips and teeth = labio/dental
  o Gums/bony ridge = alveolar ridge
  o Hard palate = palatal
  o Palatoalveolar boundary and tongue blade = palatoalveolar
  o Soft palate = velar
  o Glottis = glottal (space between the vocal folds)
■ Manner (shaping) of speech sounds
  o Stops (plosives): complete closure at some point along the vocal tract (i.e., /b/)
  o Fricatives: friction of air through a restricted opening (i.e., /f/)
  o Glides: Can be used as either vowels or consonants and are sometimes called semivowels. Involves the lips (w), the tongue (y)
  o Liquids: Can be used as either vowels or consonants and are sometimes called semivowels. Involves the tongue (l, r)

The four tables of consonants (Tables 1-1 through 1-4) are organized by manner of production, class of sound, and anatomic area. The examples are grouped into either one category or two: voiceless and voiced. Voiceless means the absence of vocal fold vibration, and voiced means the presence of vocal fold vibration. Voiced/Voiceless pairs are called Cognates which act more or less like cousins, same anatomy but one has only air through the formed space (voiceless) and one includes vocal fold vibration for pitch (voiced). These tables are a combination of those by Bunch[7] and Zemlin,[8] respectively.

Please note that the alphabetical letters for the examples use the International Phonetic Alphabet (IPA) and the examples of the sounds in parentheses are in American English. Also note in most comparison cases of voiceless and voiced examples that rhyming words are used.

The speaking habits of most people are stronger than their singing habits. Therefore, a transfer of articulatory behaviors will occur, both good and bad, from speaking into singing. The objective is to achieve a naturalness of tone quality and articulation to attain honesty of expression.

Table 1–1. Stops (plosives)		Examples	
Class of Sound	*Anatomic Area*	*Voiceless*	*Voiced*
Bilabial	Upper and lower lips	p (post)	b (boast)
Alveolar	Alveolar ridge and tongue tip	t (too)	d (do)
Palato-alveolar	Palatoalveolar ridge and tongue blade	tʃ (*ch*eap)	dʒ (*j*eep)
Velar (soft palate)	Velum and back of tongue	k (kit)	g (get)

Table 1–2. Fricatives		Examples	
Class of Sound	*Anatomic Area*	*Voiceless*	*Voiced*
Labiodental	Upper lip and teeth	f (fat)	v (vat)
Dental	Upper teeth and tongue	θ (*th*ing)	ð (*th*is)
Alveolar	Alveolar ridge and tongue tip	s (sue)	z (zoo)
Palato-alveolar	Palatoalveolar ridge and tongue blade	ʃ (*sh*e)	ʒ (be*ig*e)
Glottal	Glottis (space between the vocal folds)	h (how)	

Body/Mind/Spirit Connection

One can put into practice all the appropriate exercises but the psyche can either hinder or enhance progress. Another concept that warrants examination concerning vocal health is the understanding that each person is composed of body, mind, and spirit. When someone sings,

Table 1-3. Glides and Liquids		
Class of Sound	**Anatomic Area**	**Examples Voiced**
Bilabial	Upper and lower lips	w (we)
Palataodental	Palato-upper molars and tongue blade	y (you)
Alveolar	Alveolar ridge and tongue tip	l (let)
Palatoalveolar	Palatoalveolar ridge and tongue blade	r (red)

Table 1-4. Nasals		
Class of Sound	**Anatomic Area**	**Examples Voiced**
Bilabial	Upper and lower lips	m (me)
Alveolar	Alveolar ridge and tongue tip	n (no)
Velar	Palatoalveolar ridge and tongue blade	ŋ (ri*ng*)

all aspects of one's person are entwined. Our singing voice is our body, mind, and spirit. We cannot separate the influences of these things.[22]

Body

For a healthy singing technique, the tongue and the neck are two common elements to monitor. The tongue often gets us in trouble! The tongue is a huge structure composed of 8 to 10 muscles that are interdigitated. In fact, we can only see a small part of the tongue. We often try to control sound by controlling the position of the tongue (i.e., pulling it back too far, pressing it down in the center) instead of having the most efficient "home resting place" for the tongue tip while we are producing different vowels. Of course the tongue will have to move for consonants and change shape for vowels, but we usually overwork with pressure and manipulation of the tongue rather than simply having the efficient position of the tongue for certain consonants.

Along with the tongue, the neck is often a source of control and manipulation. A stiff and stubborn neck is a sign of the inability to manage stress. Some singers often hold it stiff with extrinsic muscle tension to feel physical control for sound in the area of the larynx. This may be done in order to psychologically "feel" control.[22]

Mind

The impulse or idea for making sound begins in the cerebral cortex of the brain.[11] The brain is the control panel or central processing unit (CPU) of our body. It sends information to all the systems that have to balance in order to sing. The singing voice is trained by the concepts that we cultivate with various exercises. Please remember that practice makes permanent and not necessarily perfect! What we practice is what becomes a learned behavior. What we dwell on is what becomes part of us.

Manipulative control often happens with the tongue, jaw, neck, or torso to psychologically "feel" voice before it can leave the mouth. Learning efficient technique and the tools to sing facilitates healthy singing. However, as one learns efficient, healthy technique, one has to get out of the way, let go and trust. Because of the need to control, manipulate, and hold to make sound happen, one must consciously let go, trust, and believe that it will happen.[22]

Spirit

What drives or motivates someone to sing? Is it a burning passion within or a desire to prove something? Is it the need for self-expression or applause? Does singing bring joy? Whatever the case may be, there is an internal reason why one chooses to sing. The essence or spirit of a person is expressed through music when they sing. If the technique is not at the level of the emotion or essence, then one will try to exert force for singing to occur. In our vocal journey we can choose to approach singing by either "make my voice be" or "allow my voice to become." As stated above, efficient technique of course aids in healthy singing. Remember, however, that singing is like faith. We have to get out of the way, let go and trust.[22]

The vocal instrument is unique and is composed of the entire person; body, mind, and spirit.[22] A singer is never able to put his or her instrument in a case. It is always with them and whenever vocalization occurs, whether laughing, screaming, crying, throat clearing, speaking, or singing, the instrument is being used. Therefore, the more knowledge a singer attains in regard to what his or her instrument is and how it is put together, the more likely the singer is able to build an efficient instrument to achieve longevity of vocal use.

Acknowledgments. The author thanks Robert O'Brien (Blue Tree Publishing) for permission to use Figures 1-1, 1-2A-C, 1-12A, B, 1-13, 1-14, 1-15, 1-16A, B, 1-17, 1-18A, B, 1-19, 1-20, 1-21, 1-22, 1-23, 1-24, 1-25, 1-26, 1-27, 1-28, 1-29, 1-30, 1-31A, B, 1-33 and 1-35.

The author thanks Chrisi Carter for permission for Figures 1-3A and B, 1-4A-C, 1-5, 1-6, 1-7, 1-8, 1-9, 1-10, and 1-11A-C.

References

1. Radionoff SL. What is the power of the voice, anyway? *Texas Sings!* 1997;Winter:8-9.
2. Radionoff SL. Warning: teaching can be hazardous to your vocal health! *Texas Sings!* 1997;Spring:19-20.
3. Radionoff SL. Command vs tools. *Texas Sings!* 2003;Fall:4-5.
4. Radionoff SL. Breath: the fundamental element of singing. *Texas Sings!* 1994;Fall:15,17.
5. Hixon TJ. *Respiratory Function in Speech and Song.* San Diego, Calif: Singular Publishing Group; 1991.
6. Sataloff RT. *Professional Voice: The Science and Art of Clinical Care.* 2nd ed. San Diego, Calif: Singular Publishing Group; 1997:111-130.
7. Bunch M. *Dynamics of the Singing Voice.* New York, NY: Springer-Verlag Wien; 1993.
8. Zemlin WR. *Speech and Hearing Science: Anatomy and Physiology.* 3rd ed. Englewood Cliffs, NJ: Prentice Hall; 1988.
9. Hirano M. *Clinical Examination of Voice.* New York, NY: Springer-Verlag Wien; 1981.

10. Sataloff RT. The human voice. *Scientific American.* 1992;December: 108–115.

11. Vincent, DJ. Personal communication, 2004.

12. Radionoff SL. How voices learn: from cognition to aesthetic experience. *Choral Journal.* 2007;47:45-53.

13. Baken RJ. An overview of laryngeal function for voice production. In: Sataloff RT, ed. *Vocal Health and Pedagogy.* San Diego, Calif: Singular Publishing Group; 1998:27–45.

14. Scherer RC. Laryngeal function during phonation. In: Rubin JS, Sataloff RT, Korovin GS, eds. *Diagnosis and Treatment of Voice Disorders.* 3rd ed. San Diego, Calif: Plural Publishing Inc; 2006:91–108.

15. Titze IR. *Principles of Voice Production.* Boston, Mass: Allyn & Bacon; 1994.

16. Titze IR. *The Myoelastic Aerodynamic Theory of Phonation.* Iowa City, IA: NCVS; 2006.

17. Pribram K. Brain mechanism in music. In: Clynes M, ed. *Music, Mind and Brain: The Neuropsychology of Music.* New York, NY: Plenum; 1982:21-35.

18. Wilson FR. *Tone Deaf & All Thumbs? An Invitation to Music Making.* New York, NY: Vintage Books; 1987.

19. Weinberger NM. Music and the brain. *Scientific American.* 2004; Nov:88–95.

20. Sundberg J. Vocal tract resonance. In: Sataloff RT, ed. *Professional Voice: The Science and Art of Clinical Care.* 2nd ed. San Diego, Calif: Singular Publishing Group; 1997:167-190.

21. Wall J, Caldwell R. *The Singer's Voice: Resonance.* Vol 4. Texas Women's University. Self-published videotape;1995.

22. Radionoff, SL. *Faith and Voice.* Portland, Ore: Inkwater Press; 2005.

Suggested Reading List

Please note that the readings in this list are not in reference format. The idea is to be able to find these via the Internet easily using the title of the book or the name of the author.

Body (Voice) Work

Alexander

The Use of the Self. FM Alexander. Orion Books. 2001.

Feldenkrais

Singing with Your Whole Self. Sam Nelson and Elizabeth Blades Zeller. Scarecrow Press. 2001.

Relaxercise. David Zemach-Bersin, Kaethe Zemach-Bersin, and Mark Reese. HarperOne. 1990.

Awareness Through Movement. Moshe Feldenkrais. HarperOne. 1991.

Linklater

Freeing the Natural Voice. Kristin Linklater. Drama Publishers. Revised 2006.

Freeing Shakespeare's Voice. Kristin Linklater. Theatre Communications Group. 1991.

Vocal Exercise Physiology

Vocal Exercise Physiology. Keith Saxon and Carole M. Schneider. Singular Publishing. 1995.

Respiration

Respiratory Function in Speech and Song. Thomas J. Hixon. Plural Publishing. 2007.

From Air to Aria: Relevance of Respiratory Behaviour to Voice Function in Classical Western Vocal Art. Monica Thomasson. Kungl Tekniska Hogskolan Publishing. 2003.

Phonation

Vocal Fold Physiology: Frontiers in Basic Science. Ed. Ingo Titze. Singular Publishing. 1993.

Vibrato. P.H. Dejonckere, Minoru Hirano,and Johan Sundberg. Singular Publishing. 1995.

The Myoelastic Aerodynamic Theory of Phonation. Ingo Titze. NCVS. 2006.

Laryngeal Function During Phonation. Scherer (Chap. 7). In *Diagnosis and Treatment of Voice Disorders*, 3rd edition, Ed. By John S. Rubin, Robert Thayer Sataloff, and Gwen S. Korovin. Plural Publishing. 2006.

Resonance Readings

Journal of Voice. New York: Raven Press.

Carlsson, G, & Sundberg, J. (1992). Formant frequency tuning in singing. Volume 6(3), 256-260.

Kent, R. D. (1993). Vocal tract acoustics. Volume 7(2), 97-117.

Miller, R., & Schutte, H. (1990). Feedback from spectrum analysis applied to the singing voice. Volume 4(4), 329-334.

Sundberg, J. (1990). What's so special about singers? Volume 4(2), 107-119.

The NATS Journal

Cleveland, T. (1992). What is formant tracking? Volume 49(1), 28-29.

Miller, R., & Franco, J. (1991). Spectrographic analysis of the singing voice. Volume 48(1), 4-5, 36.

Titze, I. (1991). What can a power spectrum tell us about the voice? Volume 47(5), 18-19.

Miscellaneous

Clinical Examination of Voice. Minoru Hirano. Springer-Verlag Wien. 1981

Professional Voice: The Science and Art of Clinical Care. Robert T. Sataloff. Raven Press. 1991.

Clinical Anatomy Made Ridiculously Simple. Stephen Goldberg. MedMaster Inc. 1984.

The Science of the Singing Voice. Johan Sundberg. Northern Illinois University Press. 1987.

Muscles: Testing and Function. Florence P. Kendall, Elizabeth K. McCreary, Patricia G. Provance. William & Wilkins. 1993.

Atlas of Human Anatomy. Frank H. Netter. CIBA-GEIGY. 1997.

Psyche/Intelligence

A Soprano on Her Head. Eloise Ristad. Real People Press. 1982.

Power Performance for Singers. Shirlee Emmons and Alma Thomas. Oxford Press. 1998.

Creating Confidence. Meribeth Bunch. Kogan Page Ltd. 1999.

The Inner Game of Music. Barry Green with Timothy Gallwey. Doubleday Press. 1986.

Frames of Mind. Howard Gardner. Basic Books 1985.

Psychology of Voice Disorders. Deborah C. Rosen and Robert T. Sataloff. Singular Publishing 1997.

Faith and Voice. Sharon L. Radionoff. Inkwater Press. 2005.

Chapter 2

How Do I "Play" It?

Vocal Technique

Introduction

Singing and sound production are about balancing the systems necessary to achieve sound for a desired outcome in the healthiest way. There are some sounds that have the potential to be harmful. For example, "grit," "growling," and glottal onsets are stylistic effects found in rock, country, and pop music. These effects must be used with the least amount of tension necessary in order to avert damage. Also, if used too often, a tension onset may become part of your technique and no longer employed just as a stylistic tool.[1] Regardless of the sound production or singing style, achieving an efficient "systems balance" in the healthiest way is the key to vocal longevity. This is what is commonly referred to as vocal technique.

Webster's Dictionary defines technique as "the method of procedure . . . in rendering an artistic work or carrying out a scientific or mechanical operation." It also defines it as "the degree of expertness in following this: as, the pianist had pleasing interpretation but poor technique" (p. 1872).[2] If we look further at the word method we find the definition "a way of doing anything; mode; procedure; process; especially a regular, orderly, definite procedure or way of teaching, investigating, etc. (p. 1134)."[2] Therefore, whether a singer studies voice with a teacher or simply "sings," he/she is training the voice via a method (intentionally or unintentionally) to create a body/voice

41

response for sound. If a person sings along with CDs or with the radio but does not take private voice lessons a CD may be the only "voice teacher" this singer has. Often singers simply mimic what they hear but don't understand how to produce it in a healthy way. Also, singers think that they can rely on what they hear internally. Unfortunately, this doesn't work because what is heard inside one's head is different than what others hear. What sounds dark and warm and powerful internally sounds manipulated and fake outside of the mouth. It is hard to get used to the internal "nonfeeling" sensation of singing. A singer will feel physical body sensation (chest, face, etc.) but the actual sound, like air, has to eventually leave the mouth. Singers are often told "you can't depend on what you hear—you have to rely on what you feel." This is true but what does it mean? If singing is supposed to have a nonfeeling or tension-free sensation how can you trust what you feel? Again, what we can trust is the process and body sensation which means paying attention to tongue position, jaw (if tense, etc.), lips, neck, hips, knees, body weight, abdomen release, among other things and not feeling sound. Generally, what we feel inside is excessive pressure internally. The process of balancing the voice (i.e., the whole body) will allow a singer to know his/her instrument and then to train the voice (body/mind/spirit) to be responsive and elastic. It is difficult to trust the process instead of trying to "make" an excellent product because the human condition is one of wanting to be in control. Singing is like golf and tennis, not power lifting. It is about the technique and follow-through not about brute force.

Let's examine an analogy of a beginning instrumentalist. If a person was a beginning trombonist, he/she would first learn the parts of the instrument. The learning process would continue as follows (1) how to put the instrument together, (2) how to hold it, (3) how to buzz into the mouthpiece, (4) how much air to blow through the instrument to create a tone, (5) how to hold the slide, (6) how to adjust the slides, and so forth. An instrumental student is taught that knowing the instrument and how to play it is the way to become excellent. This means mastering a technique by learning a method for training, not just listening to a sound and imitating it (although imitating sound is certainly part of the training). Many singers, however, are notorious for mimicking sounds and never really learn what their instrument is and how to efficiently "play" it. Inefficient technique has potential ramifications for vocal problems down the road. If the goal is healthy singing for longevity of career, then it is absolutely necessary to have efficient technique. Once one has a foundation of healthy technique, then stylism may begin.[3]

In order to have a healthy singing voice, it is important to know how to do the following: (a) Sing with healthy technique (i.e., balancing airflow, phonation, resonance, articulation, agility), (b) sing in the correct voice category/range, (c) sing in the correct tessitura (pitch area where voice comfortably sits), and (d) sing the genre (type/style) of music with the healthiest possible stylistic tools.[4]

It is my belief that the healthiest way to train as a singer is to understand the principles of how the structure (anatomy) of the voice functions to create sound (physiology). As in any other athletic endeavor, singing is a complex activity of many systems which have to balance. Working the elements with technique and healthy sound production to attain the "systems balance" must precede putting text, melody, and rhythm together all at once or immediately trying to perform a song.[3]

Sound: A Balancing Act

The act of singing can be compared to being on a teeter-totter or seesaw (Figure 2–1). The teeter-totter effect occurs when a person sitting on the ground seat pushes with their legs and is propelled into the air. Consequently, the opposite seat that was in the air goes down to the ground. Keeping the teeter-totter parallel to the ground requires a "balancing act."[5]

The shifting of power action in the teeter-totter example may be used as an analogy in regard to singing. At different times one muscle or muscle group is more active than another and a power shift takes place. Sometimes the shift is gradual and sometimes the shift is abrupt. The complex systems for sound production that interact and must be

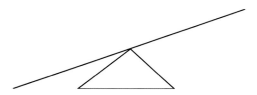

Figure 2–1. Teeter-totter.

balanced are respiration (power source), phonation (the vocal folds = raw sound source/pitch source), and resonance (the supraglottic vocal tract = the quality shaper).[5]

Basic questions to keep in mind regarding balancing the vocal system are: (a) where does the work occur, (b) what does the work, and (c) how much work has to happen? These questions may be examined in terms of pitch, loudness and articulation. A variety of muscles work together to create pitch. This chapter discusses the two most important muscles. In the most simplistic terms, the thyroarytenoid (TA) muscle shortens, and thickens the vocal fold.[6] Therefore, when lower pitches are produced the TA muscle (Figure 2-2) is active. When a higher pitch is produced the cricothyroid muscle becomes more active (Figure 2-3). The cricothyroid (CT) muscle is the principal muscle for longitudinal tension. Contraction of the CT muscle lengthens the vocal folds and thins them, which allows for a higher pitch.[7] One does not have to vocally manipulate to make pitches change because this is intrinsically how the system works![5]

In regard to loudness, when the vocal folds vibrate with greater amplitude (wider apart) there is more airflow passing through per vibration. Also, the impact or closure force of contact of the true vocal folds is greater, thereby creating a louder sound. When the

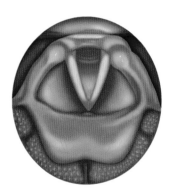

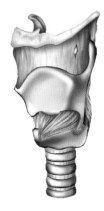

Figure 2–2. The thyroarytenoid muscle makes up the body of the true vocal folds (vocal cords).

Figure 2–3. The cricothyroid muscle runs between the cricoid and thyroid cartilages.

vocal folds vibrate closer together there is less airflow per vibration, which creates a softer sound. This is called amplitude variation and results in a change in intensity. This is perceived as a change in loudness.[6]

The basic questions asked earlier are especially pertinent to articulation. In striving to achieve precise articulation, overwork may occur in terms of jaw clenching, chewing, tongue pressure, or excessive movement of the face and lips. For example, the consonant /n/ is created by the tongue tip moving up and touching the hard palate or more specifically the alveolar ridge.[8] Frequently the tongue posture for /n/ is produced with a closed or clenched jaw. This closing and/or clenching also is often true for the production of an /l/. The tongue is a powerful muscle, and a much larger structure then often perceived (Figure 2-4). Because the tongue has an attachment to the hyoid bone, tongue tension and excessive manipulation of the tongue may lead to vocal fatigue.[5]

No matter what the style of singing, balance is the key. If longevity of voice use is a desired outcome, then knowledge and excellent use of the vocal mechanism is critical. Once again, singing and sound production are about balancing the systems necessary to achieve sound for a desired outcome in the healthiest way.[5] To achieve this, one must use exercises that will train the voice to respond. It is about using exercises that create the environment which allows for the desired response and not making or forcing the voice.

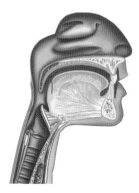

Figure 2-4. Sagittal (side) view of the resonance tract and articulators.

Exercises

Overview

The general purpose of warm-ups should be for vocal maintenance and preparation for singing. The general purpose of cool-downs is to relax the vocal system after a vigorous workout. In regard to warm-ups, often the singer begins with what should be labeled as an agility exercise (Figure 2–5). Although this is a good vocal exercise it should not sequentially be the first exercise. The sequence of preparation will make a difference in the vocal outcome.

A good preparation analogy for the singer to examine is an athlete. It would be unthinkable for a runner to put on his/her spikes, get set in the blocks, and run a 220-yard sprint prior to stretching, visualizing, and preparing the mind and body for the run ahead. Yet singers, who are vocal athletes, commit that type of error when they do not prepare the mind and body before they sing. A singer's instrument is an integration of the actual anatomic, physiologic being including the emotion and spirit. Hence, it is necessary to have time for what I call "mind-body preparation." I prefer this expression (or prep) in lieu of "warm-ups."

The activities for preparation include (1) stress release activities, (2) mental focus, and (3) mental/vocal focus. Stress release activities may include body movement such as passive or active head/neck exercises, shoulder rolls, body stretches, body movement, and relaxation exercises. Mental focus exercises should center on conscious thought of body alignment issues such as head/neck position, shoulders, upper torso, hips, knees, body weight, and so forth.[9,10] Mental/vocal focus should center on the individual singer's "systems balance" to align posture, respiration, phonation, and resonance.[9,10]

Because the singing instrument is an integration of the whole person (body/mind/spirit) it is necessary to release body and mind stress along with aligning or finding the "systems balance."

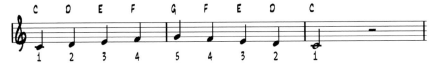

Figure 2–5. Five-note ascending/descending pattern on /ɑ/.

Exercise Flow/Organization

Stress Release Exercises

The voice can be misaligned for many reasons. It may simply be that one has just gotten up and the brain and body are not awake enough to connect at the highest level. It may also be related to external or internal stress. A certain amount of stress is normal as one goes through the rigors of life and stress can result from a variety of things. Just the pace of a busy day can create the physical reaction of stress. This reaction will cause the body to tighten and the result will be less access to airflow. Less airflow means a diminished power source and the body and voice will feel pushed by the end of the day if one does not learn how to release body and mind tension.[11] A good way to release stress and tension is to do a few repetitions of airflow management exercises—blowing air for a comfortable consistent length of time using /sh/, /wh/, /f/, or /s/ (Figure 2–6) and after blowing, release the abdominal area, let the body fill up with air, and repeat.[12] The airflow exercises are discussed in more detail later. Other stress release activities include body movement and stretching. There are many things available such as yoga and feldenkrais as mentioned in Chapter 1 along with massage and chiropractic treatments.

In regard to preparation, one might assume that because the singer has been talking since getting up then he/she is ready to sing. First, the singer may not be using healthy speech production and second, depending on the time of rehearsing, the singer may have stress which will impede the ability to achieve a full breath and affect sound production.

Relaxation/Airflow Exercises

The following exercise may be done while either sitting or lying down. Necessity for repetition will depend on the singer's stress level. It is

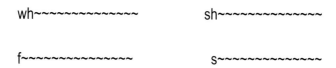

wh~~~~~~~~~~~~~~   sh~~~~~~~~~~~~~

f~~~~~~~~~~~~~~   s~~~~~~~~~~~~~~

Figure 2–6. Consonant/consonant cluster choices for airflow sounds.

often a good idea to begin this exercise while lying down on either the back or the side. If you begin in the sitting position there are already postural muscles involved which may make it more difficult to relax.

Lying Down (Figures 2–7A and 2–7B).

- Make sure that your legs are uncrossed but knees may be bent if it is more comfortable for the lower back

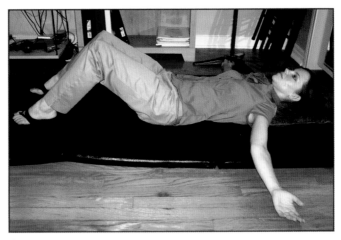

A

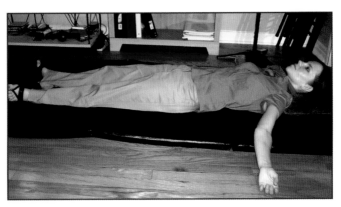

B

Figure 2–7. **A.** Prone position with bent knees for a comfortable back position. **B.** Prone position with straight legs for a comfortable back position.

■ Put a book/small pillow under your head to make sure that your posture is in line

■ Close your eyes (if you wish) and put your hands on your lower abdomen

■ Cues for body relaxation. It would be a good idea to record the body relaxation cues below:

From the top of your head to the bottom of your toes you are going to allow your body to relax. This relaxation will start at the very top of your head and move down your neck, shoulders, arms, elbows, wrists, abdomen, thighs, kneecaps, shins, ankles, and all the way out your toes (thinking /saying one word per/second).

As you are lying there, I want you to notice what happens as breath goes in and out of your body. As breath comes into your body, your body expands, and as breath leaves your body, it contracts because you no longer need that space. It's almost as if you have an inner tube that goes all the way around your body and when air comes in it fills up, and when air leaves it deflates. Abdomen and ribs (side, front, back) expand as inhalation occurs, and contract as exhalation occurs.

Sitting (Figure 2-8).

■ Make sure that your posture is in line. Lower back should not be arched—if it is then the abdominal muscles will tighten for posture and will not be available for airflow. Most often when we think of sitting up straight we hyperextend.

■ Close your eyes (if you wish) and put your hands on your lower abdomen.

■ Cues for body relaxation:

From the top of your head to the bottom of your toes you are going to allow your body to relax. This relaxation will start at the very top of your head and move down your neck, shoulders, arms, elbows, wrists, abdomen, thighs, kneecaps, shins, ankles, and all the way out your toes (thinking /saying one word per/second)

As you are sitting there, I want you to notice what happens as breath goes in and out of your body. As breath comes into your body, your body expands, and as breath leaves your body, it contracts because you no longer need that space. It's almost as if you have an inner tube that goes all the way around your body and when air

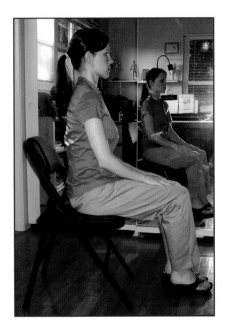

Figure 2–8. Efficient sitting position.

comes in it fills up, and when air leaves it deflates. Abdomen and ribs (side, front, back) expand as inhalation occurs, and contract as exhalation occurs.

This exercise allows for relaxation and at the same time deep airflow is being accessed. One should begin with passive airflow inhaled through either the nose or relaxed open mouth and exhaled passively using /huh/ or /wh/, and then move to a more active release of steady, managed airflow using /sh/, /s/, or /f/ (see Figure 2–6). The choice of the consonant/consonant combination /sh/, /s/, and/or /f/ creates a resistance space through which the air travels. It is what I call a "brain-ab" exercise. The steadiness of the tongue position allows for consistency of managed airflow. The objective of this exercise is to keep the volume of sound of the blowing steady from whenever one begins to whenever one ends. Steadiness is much more important than how long one is able to blow. It is about how you use the air you access, not about always achieving maximum inhalation. Furthermore, you do not always need to have a maximum inhalation. However, it is important to train the body to be able to respond for maximum inhalation should you need to use it. The desired goal is to achieve elasticity of response of the power source (respiratory system).

It is beneficial to begin in the lying down position, back and side, respectively. This is recommended because the objective is to release stress and to allow the body to function "naturally." As singing is an athletic activity, a singer takes what is "natural" to its highest level. Therefore, it is imperative to know and be aware of how the body functions before trying to have the body function at a high athletic level. Moving from the back to the side position is useful as gravity is different and one will feel more back expansion and more contraction of the abdominal muscles. It is also good because one can observe if the back muscles are pushing out near the end of the blowing out process instead of the abdominal muscles continuing to contract inward. There are pros and cons in every position. On the back gravity tends to pull everything down and back whereas the side position can make it difficult for the jaw position (gravity pulling the jaw toward the side one is lying on). It is about training for the effectiveness or efficiency of each position. When one does airflow exercises it is useful to refrain from using the terms "breathe" and "take a deep breath." There is already an association for most people with overworking to create the behavior. Remember that the objective is to "allow" not to "make," and to allow the body to function with a steady, managed airflow.

Quick Reference Guide to Blow and Relax Airflow Sequence:

- Blow out all of the air that is in you with the following sequence
  - /huh/, /wh/ relaxed passive awareness
  - /sh/, /s/, /f/ allow for more active managed release of airflow which is what one does when singing.
    - It is beneficial to repeat each consonant/consonant combination 3 to 5 times in a row. Each repetition allows the body to become more elastic thereby allowing access to more air.
    - Keep the sound volume steady from the beginning to end.
- Relax your abdomen and allow air to come in. Abdomen and ribs (side/front/back) expand as inhalation occurs.
  - Useful body positions for airflow exercises include the back, side, sitting, standing, and moving

Vocal Tension Release Exercises

The next exercise after airflow would be "vocal tension release" exercises. These consist of vocal slides using the phonemes /f and v/ in combination (beginning with the unvoiced consonant and then moving down the slide on the voiced consonant) or /shu/. The main object of these exercises is to feel the air at the front of the mouth (f/v) with ease of sound, not listening for beautiful sound. It is important to do these exercises starting in a comfortable middle range and not in the high range. First, start on a comfortable middle range pitch and slide down to a comfortable low range pitch. It should be a moderately slow glide. Be sure that the upper teeth touch the bottom lip appropriately when using the f/v combination. Airflow should be felt behind the top teeth. The teeth should touch the bottom lip at the vermilion border. If one feels the airflow coming out between the teeth then one does not have the teeth touching the bottom lip enough or there is a gap between the teeth. This exercise also may be done by using an undulating wavy slide (Figures 2–9A and B). Don't try to make exact pitch definition. Again, the important issue is a lot of air at the teeth and ease of sound. Another phoneme cluster to use is /shu/. Remember that when using /shu/ the tongue tip will not be behind the bottom teeth for the consonant cluster /sh/ but will then need to come behind the bottom teeth for the /u/ vowel. If you use the f/v combination then the tongue can be behind the bottom teeth the entire time.[11]

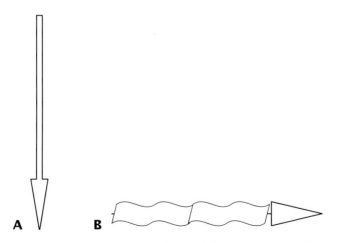

Figure 2–9. **A.** Descending slide. **B.** Wavy slide.

Descending (Crossover Airflow/Phonation/ Stretching) Exercises

The next step of preparation would be the descending APS (Airflow/ Phonation/Stretching) exercises of which there are three types. This stage connects more sound with airflow and different types of stretching without worrying about reaching or singing actual pitches. There are three basic types of slides as seen below. In regard to the vowels there is a chart for singers trained using the International Phonetic Alphabet (IPA) and a corresponding column in the chart for non-IPA user sounds (Figure 2-10).

Descending Slide—Type 1 (Figure 2-11)
- ■ This slide is a straight descending slide.
- ■ Start with a comfortable pitch and slide down.
- ■ Be sure that the tongue tip is behind the front bottom teeth the whole slide (unless you add consonants such as /l/ (see the articulation table in Chapter 1).
- ■ Be sure that the center of the tongue does not scoop or press as you go down the slide.
- ■ Consonant/vowel choices:
  - ○ **Foo, Floo
  - ○ **Foh, Flow
  - ○ **Choh, Boh, and so forth

* IPA	** Non-IPA
Fu /u/ (Food)	Foo /oo/ (Food)
Fo /o/ (Foam)	Foh /oh/ (Foam)
Flo /o/	Flow /oh/
Bum /u/ (Boom)	Boom /oo/ (Boom)
Bʌm /ʌ/	Buhm /uh/

Figure 2–10. IPA (International Phonetic Alphabet) versus non-IPA Chart.

Descending Slide—Type 2 (Figure 2-12)
- ■ This slide is a small roller coaster slide.
- ■ Start on a comfortable pitch, slide up and down a little roller coaster hill, and then slide back up and down a larger roller coaster hill (medium high).
- ■ Be sure that the center of the tongue does not scoop or press as you go down the slide.
- ■ Consonant/vowel choices:
  - ○ **Begin with Foh and change to Woh at the highest peak of the roller coaster.

Descending Slide—Type 3 (Figure 2-13)
- ■ Start with a comfortable pitch, slide down a little roller coaster hill, and then slide back up and down an even larger roller coaster hill (high).
  - ○ Males slide up through falsetto

Figure 2-11. Descending slide Type 1.

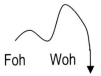

Foh   Woh

Figure 2-12. Descending slide—Type 2.

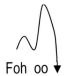

Foh oo

Figure 2-13. Descending slide—Type 3.

*IPA Vowels
**Non-IPA Vowels

- Be sure that the center of the tongue does not scoop or press as you go down the slide.
- Consonant/vowel choices:
  - **Begin with Foh and change to oo at the highest peak of the roller coaster.

Tone Balancing Exercise

The last exercise presented is called a tone balancing exercise. This consists of choosing a comfortable note in the speaking range. On a single note such as A3, Bb3, B3, or C4 for females—C4 = middle C (pitches C#4 and D4 may be used for high voice sopranos) (Figure 2-14) use the consonant vowel combination **"Boom" or **"Buhm." The object is to simply say easy repetitions of the chosen combination in slow and faster repetitions (bum-bum-bum-bum-bum). It is not necessary to push pressure forward into the /m/. Simply by choosing one of these combinations you will feel the sound move forward as /m/ is the most frontal nasal consonant. All that one does is open and close the lips for the combination.[12]

Concepts

Systems Alignment

Mental focus should center on body alignment issues such as jaw position, tongue position, head/neck position, shoulders, upper torso, hips, knees, body weight, and so forth (see Chapter 1 for more detail).[9] This type of focus may be achieved during many different exercises. One way to accomplish this would be to have a visual checklist to glance at while carrying out an exercise. It may feel like one is thinking too hard, or too much about technique at first. However, it is by repetitive

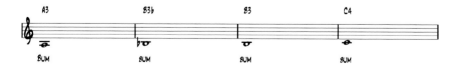

Figure 2–14. Tone balancing pitches for females.

behavior and thought of the principles that guide efficient function of the vocal system that allow for mastering a healthy technique. Things in the checklist of items to pay attention to may include:

Quick Reference Guide to Systems Alignment:

■ posture/body alignment
   ○ i.e., Head/neck position, shoulders, and so forth (Chapter 1).
■ airflow
   ○ Freely flowing or impeded? (See checklist Chapter 4)
■ phonation
■ resonance
   ○ chamber consistency
   ○ articulation
      • See separation technique (later section this chapter)

Building Block Approach

The singer can prioritize the mental/vocal focus during the building block exercises. Singing is like building a house. When building a house, the foundation comes first, then the walls and the roof follow before work begins on the inside. As in building a house, there is a logical sequence when creating sound. Airflow management is the foundation (the respiratory system = power source), phonation (pitch source) the walls, and resonance (sound shaper) the roof. After you have layered these three systems then you can begin to work on agility, strength, and musicianship along with interpretation and style. An example of the building block approach would be the following: (1) begin with airflow on /sh/, /f/, or /s/, (2) next add phonation on a single note using /shu/, /fu/, or /su/, and (3) last add resonance by adding an /m/ to the previous phonation /shum/, /fum/, or /sum/ and repeat the pattern (shum-mum-mum) (Figure 2–15).

There is a direct link between the first step, airflow, to the second step, phonation. The same consonant/consonant combination for the respiratory mechanics of airflow begins both steps and then we add vocal fold vibration for the second step. Likewise, by adding the /m/ for resonance, the third step starts the same as the second step but allows for frontal directionality for the resonance. As /m/ is the most frontal nasal consonant (as previously mentioned), it is not necessary to press or push air pressure forward. One simply closes the lips and the airflow travels forward toward the lips. After the basic sound has been balanced then agility of vocal fold lengthening and shortening may be attempted. A desirable way to begin is to use small patterns so that a singer will not fight against self for control. The numbers used to define these patterns below are based on a major scale (Figure 2–16). These patterns are 1-7-1, 1-2-1, and 3-2-1. These patterns may be added together to gradually increase the range of agility such as: 1-7-1-2-1, 1-2-1-7-1, 3-2-1-7-1, and so on (Figure 2–17A).[12]

Skipping patterns (Figure 2–17B). Notice that these start from top down and then alternate. It is usually more accessible to start with a stretch and release than to go in the opposite direction. This is especially hard when working on extremes of the range. The same procedure for the thirds and fourths can be carried out for wider skips (Figure 2–17C).

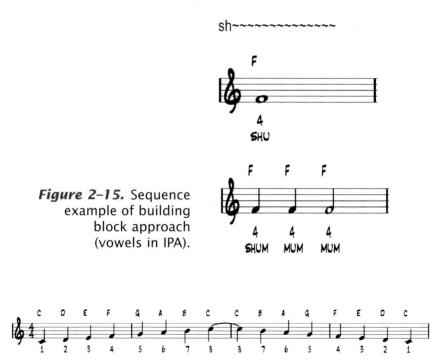

Figure 2–15. Sequence example of building block approach (vowels in IPA).

Figure 2–16. Major scale with traditional notation.

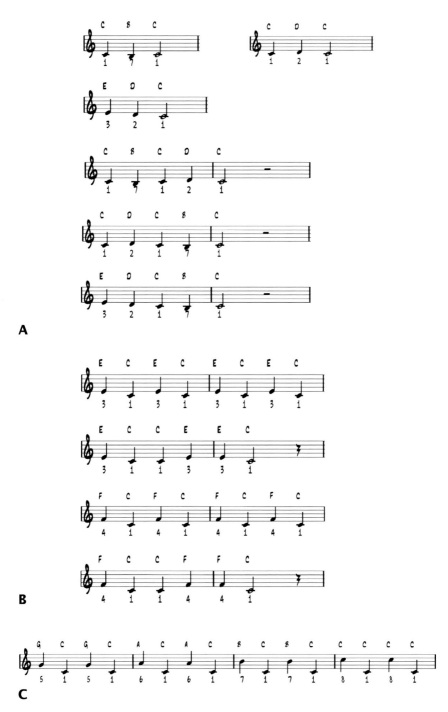

Figure 2-17. **A.** Series of small patterns. **B.** Skipping patterns.
C. Wider skips.

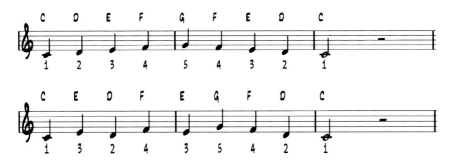

Figure 2-18. Agility exercises.

Agility exercises (Figure 2-18). These are but a few examples. There are many good books that have been written that may be used such as Viardot, Marchesi, Vaccai, and others.

Quick Reference Guide to Patterns:

■ Begin with small patterns
  - 1-7-1
  - 1-2-1
  - 3-2-1
■ Number of repetitions
  - Each pitch area for a pattern should be repeated 3 to 5 times to create consistency of the systems behavior
■ Increase the range and agility of the patterns
  - Add the above patterns together
  - 1-7-1-2-1, 1-2-1-7-1, 3-2-1-7-1
  - Add skipping patterns
  - Add longer scalar patterns

Multitasking Exercises

The purpose of the following exercises is to combine kinesthetic response with sound. These exercises are a precursor to adding sound to choreography. The following sequence may be used in progression. Below the sound production variables are listed first.

- Airflow
- Single note long tone
- Single note rhythmic variation
- 3- to 4-note pitch variation
  - With single consonant/vowel combination
  - With text (songs)
- Phrase of song
  - With single consonant/vowel combination
- Text of song
  - chanting on a single note
- Text + melody

Next, add the following kinesthetic body movements to the above parameters. Notice that the following physicality starts with a simple activity and progresses to a higher level of complexity.

- Arm movement
- Body sway
- Body pattern
- Actual choreography

As mentioned earlier in the pattern exercises, it is important to repeat each item that you do 3 to 5 times in order to allow for consistency to occur.

Styles

Balance and alignment of the vocal instrument, composed of the body/mind/spirit connection, is just the beginning for the performer. If one knows where center point is, then one can experiment with how far one may go from the central balance point for coloration and effect and still have integrity of technique. It really does not matter what style of music someone sings. What truly matters is what the balance point of the voice is. If a singer knows his/her balance point, then he/she will be able to experiment with breath, resonance (e.g., nasalance), articulation, straight tone, and delayed vibrato (along with other aspects) for coloration and effect. It is no different than a painter having a palate with many colors to choose from to create nuance in his or her painting.

In regard to vocal styles and stylistic tools, there are many vocal sounds that can be made and some sounds have the potential to be harmful. For example, "grit," "growling," and glottal onsets are stylistic effects found in rock, country, and pop music. These tools must be used with the least amount of tension needed to avert damage. Also, if used too often, a tension onset may become part of one's technique and no longer employed just as a stylistic tool.[1] These habits often creep into the speaking voice adding to the harmful effects. It is possible to create a desired vocal tool (i.e., grit, growl) in more than one way. The key to longevity of career is finding and understanding the "systems balance" and alignment for singing before creating stylism. Balance must be attained before power, agility, or style. This analogy can be clearly seen in sports. For example, take a gymnast. It makes sense that a gymnast stretches and finds his/her center of gravity first, whether it be on the balance beam or floor exercise, before doing any flips, turns, or difficult combinations. One might consider a gymnast foolhardy if he/she were to attempt difficult movements before balancing the body and mind. Singers, however, are notorious for ignoring balance and head immediately to agility, power, and style. They even attempt to "warm up" by singing what they consider to be an easy song. There are so many variables to be aligned that it is critical for the voice professional to find his/her systems balance and alignment.[11]

Characterization

When creating a character for performance, a singer should always develop the character and body movement within the framework of his or her physical parameters. This will include things such as height, flexibility, mobility, arm span, and so forth. Other factors to consider include interpretation of the text and delivery. Also it will be important to give the illusion of an emotion such as anger, without actually becoming angry to the point of losing the center point of the vocal balance. This is especially important when a singer has to portray more than one character in a show.

Learning New Music

When we process and learn various bits of information there are often systems of symbols and shapes such as letters or numbers. These are the fundamentals we build on. In learning music there are fundamental patterns of rhythms and sounds that we must understand, recognize, and be able to duplicate. The fundamentals function as the groundwork toward the goal of a musical experience. To be able to shift from cognition to replication to musicality and aesthetic experience is the aspiration. Music reading, efficient practice of the music, and healthy voice use are necessary to reach this objective.[3]

Music Learning Methods

Learning by Rote

Most of us are familiar with learning by rote. Someone does something and we copy what is done. This is called rote or learning by imitation. Eminent music educator Edwin Gordon likens this method to using tracing paper to copy a picture.[13] The method of learning by imitation is basic and primary to life in general, and is widely used in elementary music programs, by voice teachers, choir directors, and singers alike. Often it seems that imitation is the fastest way to get the job done whether it is for learning of parts or example of expression. One of the drawbacks of learning by rote is that a person has to rely on his/her memory for accuracy. Problems can occur with this when there is no written record of what has been taught for the person to reference. However, that being said, learning by rote can be advantageous for ear training and system memory (learning to vocally and aurally recognize patterns). It can also feel more like one is playing a game rather than working hard to get it right. We give ourselves permission to just "do" rather than tell ourselves that something is difficult. If one does begin with imitation one hopes that he/she will move to audiation. Gordon defines audiation as "when one hears *and comprehends* music silently, the sound of the music no longer being or never having been physically present" (p. 25).[13] Two researchers conducted an interesting study. They scanned the brains of nonmusicians who either listened to music or imagined hearing the same piece of music. It was found that many of the same areas in the temporal lobes were activated in either case.[14]

Traditional Staff Notation

Music reading with traditional staff notation is a skill that has been taught in music education dating back to the original colonies.[15] Traditional notation demands learning many different variables to use as decoding skills before it can effectively be used as a reading tool. For reading staff notation solfege may be used (movable or fixed do), note names may be used, and numbers that correspond to the eight-note scale may be used. The goal is to attain the level of audiation regardless of the method used. Traditional notation takes the guess work out of singing. It is also a type of shorthand transcription for a musical idea that can be replicated or duplicated by anyone which can then be personally interpreted. One drawback in traditional notation is that many spots on a page (i.e., many sixteenth notes) can look difficult and may predispose one to tensing up prior to singing.[3]

Nashville Number System

Along with traditional notation there is also the Nashville Number System (NNS) for understanding and transcribing music for performance. This system emerged in the late 1950s and was originated by Neal Matthews, a member of the "Jordanaires."[16] It is a method of substituting Arabic numerals for melody notes, as well as Arabic numerals for traditional Roman numeral chords (i.e., 1 4 5 instead of I IV V). This method, however, does not dismiss learning basic theory of keys, scales, and rhythms on the part of the musician. In this system the numbers 1 to 7 are used in scale relationship and arrows are used to denote up and down (along with other NNS decoders). Figure 2-19 shows the scale used with the Nashville Number System. Figure 2-20 shows how this is applied to the first line of the melody "Joy to the World."[3]

The method that one uses to learn new music, whether rote, traditional notation, or the NNS may well have a bearing on (a) the rate of learning, (b) the amount of new knowledge one is able to learn, and (c) how independent versus dependent one is in regard to learning. Regardless of the method of learning, pattern recognition

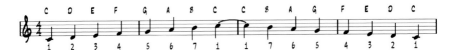

Figure 2-19. Major scale with Nashville Number System (NNS).

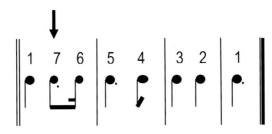

Figure 2-20. "Joy to the World" opening melody using the NNS.

and duplication is the goal of the fundamentals. Reimer calls this functional literacy.[15] This skill must be reached first before musicality and interpretation can take place.[3]

Efficient Practice

Basic Elements of a Song

When beginning to learn a song the broad elements to be examined include: (a) key(s) of the song, (b) meter signature(s), and (c) recurring sections. Next, a further analysis would consist of breaking down the song into its basic elements in regard to melody. It is crucial for students to recognize what I call "recurring melodic patterns." In deconstructing a song, it is helpful to consider that melodies are made up of phrases, which are made of patterns joined together, which are made of intervals joined together, which are single pitches joined together.[3]

Recognition of patterns is vitally important in learning songs. Our brains actually go through an "editing" process to look for things that are different.[17] Therefore, if we already have a library of patterns to draw upon, there is a foundation for linking familiar to familiar which allows for quicker progress toward identification of what is different or novel.[3]

Recurring Melodic Patterns

Recurring melodic patterns may be used as preparation for patterning the ears, brain, and larynx prior to singing the song. The process is as follows:

- pick out recurring melodic patterns to use as exercises,
- break them down into small patterns (3 to 4 notes)—don't use an entire phrase
- write these out on manuscript paper
  - It is easiest to write the pattern in C (major and parallel minor). As it will be used as a vocalise it is not necessary to write it in a more complex key.
- choose a comfortable consonant/vowel combination
- for consonant choices begin with either an /m/ /w/ /sh/ /b/ or /p/
  - for rationale see Chapter 4
- for vowel choices start with /u/ or /o/
  - for rationale see Chapter 4
- start in a comfortable range and then move the pattern up and down by half steps
- change consonant/vowel combination
- add one of the vowels found in the actual music of the melodic pattern chosen
- add all of the actual vowels to the consonant chosen from above.[3]

The foundation for patterns to be built upon will be the major scale shown earlier. The major scale is referenced with the numbers 1 to 8 (1) (see Figure 2-16).[3] It is of note to mention that if the pattern 8-7-6-5 is superimposed over 4-3-2-1 one can see that both patterns have the same intervallic relationship, half step - whole step - whole step. Therefore, it is not necessary to refer to 8-7-6-5 but only to 4-3-2-1, the most basic intervallic relationship pattern.

How are recurring melodic patterns found? Let's begin by examining a common carol. In Figure 2–21, the first words "Joy to the world" use the pattern 4321 but the next words "the Lord is come" also use

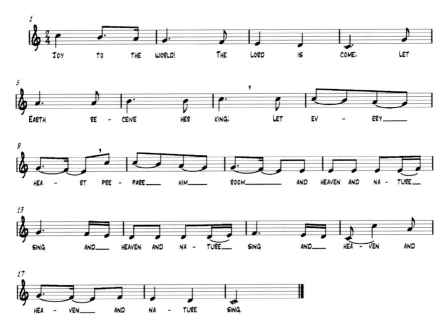

Figure 2–21. Joy to the World (verse 1).

a 4321 pattern. Again, if the relationship of a key is used then the first 4321 could be called 8765. Nevertheless, it still acts in interval relationship as a 4321 pattern. Therefore, the pattern 4321 may be practiced as a vocalise (exercise) up and down the scale to solidify the brain/body patterning for the system of phonation (Note: when recurring patterns are used it is not necessary to write down on manuscript paper the occurrence of a pattern that happens in different pitch areas as they will be used up and down the scale as a vocalise). The 4321 pattern is also used in ascending order in measures 4 to 7 "let earth receive her King."[3]

Recurring Melodic Patterns in "Joy to the World." All the recurring patterns in "Joy to the world" will be written as if in the key of C (Major and parallel minor). The pattern 4-3-2-1 (Figure 2–22A) is found in the following measures:

■ one and two with the text "Joy to the world"
■ two, three, and four with the text "the Lord is come,"

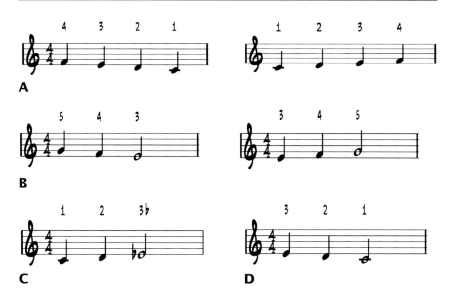

Figure 2–22. **A.** Recurring pattern 4 3 2 1 / 1 2 3 4. **B.** Recurring pattern 5 4 3 / 3 4 5. **C.** Recurring pattern 1 2 3 flat. **D.** Recurring pattern 3 2 1.

- four to seven in ascending order with the text "Let earth receive her King,"
- seven and eight with the text "Let every"
- nine and ten with the text "prepare Him."[3]

The pattern 5-4-3 (Figure 2–22B) is found in the following measures:

- nine with the text "heart"
- with the text "room,"
- 15 and 16 with the text "and hea(ven)
- The ascending order of this pattern is found in measures 11, 12, and 13 with the text "And Heaven and nature sing."

The pattern 1-2-3 flat (Figure 2–22C) is actually heard in the repeat of the sequence "heaven and nature sing" in measures 14 and 15. Arguments could be made for this pattern to be called a 4-3-2 by adding "and heaven and nature sing" and then repeating this in a mirrored ascending pattern. However, the pitches for "and" in measure 14 act more like passing notes to the next sequential pattern.

The pattern 3-2-1 (Figure 2–22D) is found in the following measures:

■ 15 and 16 with the text "and hea(ven)
■ 18 and 19 with the text "nature sing."

One might ask why the word "and" was not added to this sequence to create the 4-3-2-1 pattern. The reason is much the same as above; that the pitch for "and" acts like a neighboring tone (upper neighbor to be exact).

It would also be relevant to practice the minor 6th interval from mm. 9 and the octave jump in mm. 16. Although these intervallic jumps do not recur within the verse they will recur as each successive verse is sung. As is seen from this analysis of patterns, "Joy to the World" is based on four main patterns.[3]

When phrases are broken down into smaller repetitive patterns it actually boils the melody down into its most basic form. There are a finite number of patterns in an eight-note scale, and a finite number of ways these patterns are joined together. These patterns will be revisited in many songs.[3]

It is also a beneficial practice to include recurring rhythmic patterns and/or difficult rhythmic patterns during the preparation or warm-up time. In "Joy to the World" a potential rhythm to practice for clarity would be the beginning rhythm with the dotted figure seen in Figure 2–23.[3]

Separation Technique

Another concept for efficient practice is the "Separation Technique." This means to separate the elements of a song such as rhythm of the melody, the melody tones, and the text. Rhythm is the most fundamental element of music. To begin, count or clap the rhythm of the melody. It would be advantageous to clap the melody rhythm along with the accompaniment. If you are unable to play the accompani-

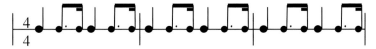

Figure 2–23. Recurring rhythmic pattern.

ment or do not have a rehearsal accompanist, have someone record the accompaniment and clap the melody along with the recorded accompaniment. Depending on how the accompaniment and the melody rhythm fit together, it can be difficult and the accompaniment can pose a problem with accuracy. It would also be helpful to add count singing.[3]

Consider how a rhythmic variation of the four-note pattern, 4-3-2-1, can totally change a song. It is interesting to observe that when the first four notes of the carol are played from Figure 2–24, the carol is immediately recognized, almost without fail.

In Figure 2–25, the meter has changed from duple to triple and the pattern is used in both descending and ascending order. There is also use of a descending skip of a perfect 4th.

This next example is simply a repetitive descending 4-3-2-1 (Figure 2–26).

In Figure 2–27, notice that the triplet feel is used along with the notes being in ascending order.

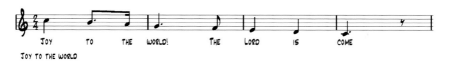

Figure 2–24. First line of the carol "Joy to the World."

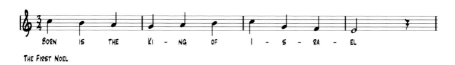

Figure 2–25. Middle section of the carol "The First Noel."

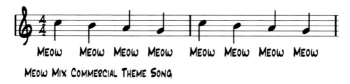

Figure 2–26. TV commercial.

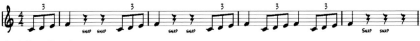

ADAM'S FAMILY THEME SONG

Figure 2–27. TV theme song.

In regard to melody it is important to study the melody without the text added. Ideally it would be excellent if a singer had the ability to play his/her part on the piano (this is an excellent ear training exercise). When learning a new song, working text and melody together has the potential to cause confusion. It would also be of benefit to listen to the melody—CAUTION—do not listen for sound production if listening to another singer. It is constructive to learn the notes by replacing the actual text with a comfortable consonant/vowel combination such as /mum/ /mIm/ /mo/ /mu/ /shu/ /wo/ /wu/ /bu/ /bo/ /fo/ or /flo/. When working on a song, singers need to take into consideration thinking about terms such as ease, freedom, and approach versus "hitting" a note or "pounding" out a part. If singers vocally and mentally approach learning a song with effortful words in mind what is the behavioral association? Hitting, pounding, and banging of notes can have a negative influence in the approach of vocal production and the systems balance (airflow, phonation, resonance).[3]

In regard to the text, it is important to work the articulation so that one can focus on the movable articulators (lips, tongue, jaw) to check for any excessive effort. Begin to work on the text with the following system:

- chant the text of the song on a single pitch—first not in rhythm—second time in rhythm
- write text on index cards for memorization (use as flash cards)
- type out text on a single sheet to use as a monologue (can also aid in memorization)
- research and discuss interpretation[3]

Putting It Together

Finally, put the song together with the musical elements of rhythm, melody, and text. After the song elements have been combined then it is appropriate to work the song for both musicianship and textual interpretation. Often when reading a new song a singer sings through the song one or two times with music and text together and by the third time is trying to make it a "performance."

Singing a song is a creative, complex process that combines the "balancing act" of tone production along with the basic elements of a song as discussed above. Consider the following issues of phonation. In singing a melody there is a constant shifting of the lengthening and shortening of the vocal folds for pitch change. There is also a changing of the thickness of the edge that vibrates depending on the pitch and the register. When musicianship comes into play (i.e., crescendo = loud, diminuendo = soft, etc.) there is a shifting of the amount of airflow per wave cycle and force of closure shifting that occurs. When considering the text the main factors to be dealt with are articulation and interpretation. In articulation we must consider efficient production of the text along with potential necessary modifications. When taking into account the elements involved in learning and singing a song, there are many bits of information for the brain to decipher and decode.[3]

Rehearsal Techniques. After all of the preliminary wood shedding and preparation from working recurring melodic patterns and use of the separation technique, one is ready to practice phrases and sections. When the song is put back together, there are areas that will arise that need cleanup. Be sure to work sections. Don't just sing through the whole song over and over—practice makes permanent—not perfect! If there is an area that is difficult, put the pattern, phrase or section into a comfortable pitch area and take it up and down by half-step. Also choose a comfortable consonant/vowel combination as discussed in previous exercises.

In addition, it is beneficial to run through a song from start to finish with different priorities in mind. Use both a technical run and a performance run. During the technical run concentrate on the issues of "mental focus" as discussed earlier. During the performance run the objective is to add the musicality and interpretation of performance. After the performance run, take the time to think about and analyze how much excellence of technique transferred into the performance.

Accompaniment Choices. Finally, a note needs to be inserted about working with different accompaniment situations. There are pros and cons when working with a live accompaniment of some kind (piano, band, etc.) as well as a recorded track or practice tape/CD.

Live—Pros and Cons:

■ Pro = can have an interplay or dialogue musically with the accompaniment for interpretation.

■ Con = scheduling rehearsals can prove to be difficult sometimes and can be expensive depending on the number of people involved.

Recorded Track—Pros and Cons:

■ Pro = can practice with the music whenever it is convenient.

■ Con = you are stuck within the parameters of the already recorded variable of tempo and musicality choices.

Conclusion

The foundation of healthy singing is a solid consistent technique based on the structure (anatomy) and function (physiology) of how the voice works. This must be built with exercises that train the voice (body/mind/spirit) to be responsive and elastic. This means mastering a technique by learning a method for training and not simply mimicking sounds. It is critical to attain a "systems balance" prior to stylizing or creating a character. In order for the most efficient learning to occur, a logical flow or organization of exercises is suggested. Just as in other endeavors that use the body, there needs to be a preparation time prior to becoming more athletic. It is also important to start with small patterns and then build to longer scalar and skipping patterns to increase agility. Also for those involved in stage performance, multitasking exercises are beneficial.

A singer must have knowledge of healthy voice production as well as musical knowledge to be able to analyze and separate the various elements that need practice prior to putting a song together. Bennett Reimer provides nice clear-cut definitions of *analysis* as coming from the Greek word to "loosen up" and *confusion* which essentially means "fused together." Analysis allows us to separate how things work to combat confusion. It is important to dissect things, but Reimer cautions that after dissection we must not leave things picked apart and in disarray but learn to use evaluation and then put things back together.[15]

Learning new music whether by rote, traditional staff notation, or the Nashville Number System is a means to an end, that of creating a musical experience. How does the method of choice for reading and learning music affect the voice? It has been my experience as both an observer and participator that singers try to do too much at one time with whatever method they choose. When the mental focus is divided among too many variables at one time problems can occur both musically and vocally. Therefore, the practice tool of working on recurring melodic patterns and recurring rhythmic patterns along with the separation technique is highly recommended.[3]

When putting it all together, (voice, song, interpretation) keep in mind that there are many variables involved as well as the many interactive systems that balance. When problems arise during rehearsal, remember to separate variables for cleanup such as melody and text and use both technical and performance runs of songs. Last, be aware that there are pros and cons of accompaniment choice for rehearsal.

Acknowledgments. The author thanks Robert O'Brien (Blue Tree Publishing) for permission to use Figures 2-2, 2-3, and 2-4. The author thanks Chrisi Carter for permission for Figures 2-7A, 2-7B, and 2-8.

References

1. Radionoff SL, Binkley CK. *Commercial Singing for Classical Singers.* Professional workshop presented at The Voice Foundation's 25th Annual Symposium Care of the Professional Voice, Philadelphia, Pa; June 1996.
2. Webster N, McKechnie J. *Webster's New Twentieth Century Dictionary Unabridged.* New York, NY: Simon and Schuster; 1983.
3. Radionoff SL. How voices learn: From cognition to aesthetic experience. *Choral Journal.* 2007;47:45-53.
4. Garrett JD, Radionoff SL, Rodriguez M, Stasney CR. *Vocal Health.* Lynnewood, Wash: Blue Tree Publishing; 2003.
5. Radionoff SL. Sound: a balancing act. *Texas Sings!* 2005;Winter:8-9.
6. Sataloff RT. *Professional Voice: The Science and Art of Clinical Care.* 2nd ed. San Diego, Calif: Singular Publishing Group; 1997:111-130.
7. Baken RJ. An overview of laryngeal function for voice production. In: Sataloff RT, ed. *Vocal Health and Pedagogy.* San Diego, Calif: Singular Publishing Group; 1998:27-45.
8. Bunch M. *Dynamics of the Singing Voice.* New York, NY: Springer-Verlag Wien; 1993.
9. Radionoff SL. Warning: Teaching can be hazardous to your vocal health. *Texas Sings!* 1997;Spring:19-20.

10. Radionoff SL. What is a warm-up and what is it for? *Texas Sings!* 2004;Winter:8–9.
11. Radionoff SL. Artistic vocal styles and technique. In: Benninger MS, Murray T, eds. *The Performer's Voice.* San Diego, Calif: Plural Publishing Inc; 2006:51–59.
12. Radionoff SL. The music educator: a high-risk professional voice. In: Stemple JC, ed. *Voice Therapy Clinical Studies.* 2nd ed. San Diego, Calif: Singular Publishing Group; 2000:397–409.
13. Gordon EE. *A Music Learning Theory for Newborn and Young Children.* Chicago, Ill: GIA Publications, Inc; 2003.
14. Weinberger NM. Music and the brain. *Scientific American.* 2004;Nov: 88–95.
15. Reimer B. *A Philosophy of Music Education.* Englewood Cliffs, NJ: Prentice Hall; 1989.
16. Williams C. *The Nashville Number System.* Nashville, Tenn: Self-published; 2005.
17. Pribram K. Brain mechanism in music. In: Clynes M, ed. *Music, Mind and Brain: The Neuropsychology of Music.* New York, NY: Plenum; 1982:21–35.

Chapter 3

How Do I Take Care of It?

Arts Medicine and Professional Voice Care

In 1987, a new specialty in the field of medicine began to be established. This new métier, arts medicine, offers specialized treatment for singers, dancers, piano and string performers, visual artists, and others; and most of the new treatment sites, Arts Medicine Centers, are located in large metropolitan areas. The first textbook for arts medicine, *Textbook of Performing Arts Medicine*, was published in 1991 to help establish this new trend.[1]

At the same time, a new subspecialty within the field of otolaryngology, professional voice care, was emerging. Before further discussion can proceed, it is necessary to define who belongs in the category of the professional voice user. Voice professionals are those whose livelihood depends on their voices. There is some difference of opinion in this field as to the population that describes professional voice users. Certainly most agree that singers and actors are professional voice users, as by definition they depend on their voices for their livelihood: but what about music teachers? The music teacher without a voice would be out of a job. All music teachers depend on their voices for their livelihood. In fact, many other professions such as sales people, lawyers, professors, and so forth depend on their voices for their livelihood. The Voice Foundation (founded in 1969)[2] located in Philadelphia, Pennsylvania uses the title Care of the Professional Voice when organizing its annual symposium.

Dr. Robert T. Sataloff published the first article devoted to care of the professional voice in 1981.[3] The groundwork for this new subspecialty actually began over 30 years ago with the inception of the Voice Foundation's Annual Symposium on Care of the Professional Voice.

This symposium, begun by Dr. Wilbur James Gould in 1972, was the catalyst of an international interdisciplinary education for laryngologists, voice scientists, speech-language pathologists, singing teachers, and singers[2,3] as well as nutritionists, and body movement specialists. In 1991 Dr. Sataloff also published the first textbook devoted entirely to professional voice care entitled: *Professional Voice: The Science and Art of Clinical Care*.[4] In order to better understand the interdisciplinary nature of this profession, it is of benefit to briefly examine two interrelated fields which are intertwined in Professional Voice Care: Vocal Pedagogy and Voice Science.

Interrelated Field: Vocal Pedagogy

Chapter 2 stated that whether a singer studies voice with a teacher or simply sings, he/she is training the voice via a method (intentionally or unintentionally) to create a body/voice response for sound. A voice teacher (pedagogue) is known to primarily teach technique whereas a vocal coach focuses on the repertoire and acting/interpretive elements of songs. Webster's Dictionary defines pedagogy as "the art or science of teaching; especially the instruction in teaching methods" (p. 1320).[5]

A vocal pedagogue's (voice teacher) job is to give a singer the tools and methodology to train the voice to respond with a (one hopes, healthy and efficient) technique that will allow one to sing whatever genre (style) of music that one wishes to sing. When studying with a voice teacher, there is a built-in outside monitor who will watch and listen to how one produces sound. However, don't expect the voice teacher to do all of the work. It is the teacher's job to provide the tools necessary for the singer to achieve vocal production in the healthiest manner possible but it is the singer's job to use the tools given.

Mirrors don't lie! Mirror practice is an excellent way to self-monitor whether in the vocal studio or in a practice room (Figure 3–1). As the voice teacher cannot always be present, mirror practice will allow for self-monitoring to aid the singer in healthy vocal production. Furthermore, what often feels "natural" may be habitual and looking into a mirror will help the singer distinguish the difference between what "feels natural" and what the anatomy is doing. Another self-monitor system is audio or videotaping lessons or practice sessions. If the

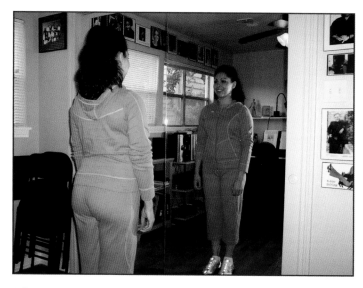

Figure 3–1. Mirror practice for self-monitoring.

singer is able to trust that the recording will capture his or her sound then he or she will be able to let go of the desire to monitor with his/her ears while singing. This will aid in the awareness of what is felt as opposed to what is heard. This mode of monitoring becomes even more important when the singer no longer has the consistent benefit of outside observers such as a voice teacher or vocal coach.[6]

History

Prominent writings on the art, craft, and science of the teaching of singing can be traced to the 1700s and represent various methods of teaching singing. In *Historical Vocal Pedagogy Classics*, Coffin[7] outlines the methods of prominent pedagogues such as Pier Francesco Tosi, Giambattista Mancini, Manuel García I, and Manuel García II. Included are a number of other early pedagogical methods by Mathilde Marchesi, Julius Stockhausen, and Lilli Lehmann. It is interesting to note that Marchesi and Stockhausen, who became known as great teachers, were students of Manuel García II.[8,9]

One of the most eminent schools of vocal pedagogy is the *bel canto* school, which can be traced from Nicola Porpora (1686–1768) through the García family. The *bel canto* school is the Italian school of singing which means "beautiful singing." There is no description of what Porpora taught other than the music that he wrote for his students. The first important writing on the teaching of singing was published in 1723 by Tosi.[7] Although there are different schools of teaching,[10] the influence of the *bel canto* school is evident in the German school of pedagogy through García's teaching of Johanna Wagner (Richard Wagner's niece) and Julius Stockhausen.[8,9]

Reid, who was a prominent pedagogue in the 1950s and 1960s, believed that scientific studies by García and others were partially responsible for the decline of the *bel canto* school and that the information "clouded" tone production.[11] Coffin refutes this statement and asserts that "there is no better understanding of the *bel canto* school than through García" (p. 206).[7,9]

In defining his school of vocal training, Reid delineates the *bel canto* school as being a psychological method as opposed to the application of science to voice training. He states that "in making a choice between scientific application to voice training and the psychological method of the early teachers of *bel canto*, it is important to remember that one is dealing with a muscular organization" (p. 46).[9,11]

This viewpoint, which states that *bel canto* was purely a psychological method, is incorrect in light of further historical review. Miller quotes the study of acoustic adjustments by Mancini in 1774: "If the harmony of . . . the mouth and 'fauce' is perfect, then the voice will be clear and harmonious. But if these organs act discordantly, the voice will be defective, and consequently the singing spoiled" (p. 375).[12] Further scientific interest is seen in a description of respiration in singing by Jean-Baptiste Berard from 1775:

> . . . the ribs raise outwardly, and . . . the diaphragm . . . descends and compresses the abdomen. . . . For good expiration . . . air must be made to leave with more or less force, with more or less volume, according to the character of the song (p. 375).[9,12]

Along with Reid, Stanley was another prominent pedagogue in the 1950s; each published a voice book in 1951. Whereas Reid's book defined his school of functional voice training, Stanley's publication was scientific. A review was published in the August, 1951 issue of *Musical Courier*. The reviewer states that:

. . . the books might have been written, respectively, by a man from Mars and a man from Venus, so radically different are the vocal philosophies behind them . . . Reid seems to know what he is talking about—but so, also, does Stanley. Whom to believe? The proof should lie in the pudding—but here again neither of the two, as far as this writer knows, has produced a pupil that would come anywhere near the claims each sets forth for his teaching principles. And when one gets through reading these two books, each excellent in its way one still has no idea why singing today is in the wretched state it is (p. 28).[9,13]

It seems that not much has changed today. There are still many methods and pedagogues that push their self-named/proclaimed method. The reality is that the singing voice is built on the anatomy and physiology of a singer's body. Let's stop arguing about the "so-and-so method" and truly get to the basics of how the body works to produce sound! All musicians need to learn about their instrument so that they can take care of it. Singers are not exempt from this; in fact, it is even more important as there are so many changing variables involved.

Reid further states that García's motivation behind the invention of the laryngoscope was a desire to obtain a shortcut to achieving vocal mastery.[11] This view by Reid must be questioned, however, in light of a review of Part I of García's *A Complete Treatise on the Art of Singing*. García states that no vocalises are found in this work. He discusses in further detail that they were excluded from this method because they no longer have the previous advantage of the complete development of the resources of the voice but, instead, cause problems. A lengthy footnote was added, much of which merits quotation:

> Formerly, in the teaching of solfege (la solmisation), the master, by careful precautions, would prevent in advance all the faulty habits which might have been able to prejudice the future studies of the singer. . . . Today the study of music and that of singing are no longer confided to the same master, and the first of these studies is only the incomplete or faulty preparation for the second (p. xviii).[9,14]

Contemporary vocal pedagogue, Richard Miller, defines two important objectives for the studio voice teacher. He states that the contemporary voice teacher's studio teaching objectives should be based on the following two points: (1) to analyze vocal problems and

(2) to design proper solutions for them. He states that the main goal of the voice teacher should be to do no harm and that:

> ... every aspect of vocal technique must be in agreement with what is known about healthy vocal function. . . . Above all, as teachers of singing in a scientific age, we must ask ourselves how much we really know about the subject matter we deal with. Do we have facts, or do we rely on anecdotal opinions? Do we know the literature of our own field, as well as that of related fields (p. 380)? [9,12]

Interrelated Field: Voice Science

History

Though important pedagogical writings about the voice can be traced to the 1700s, scientific writings about the voice date back centuries earlier. In fact the cultural history of the larynx and voice dates back to more than 2,000 years before the birth of Christ. Hans von Leden, eminent laryngologist and father of phonosurgery, describes four cultural phases that the concept of voice production passed through: stage one the fictitious or mythical stage, stage two the metaphysical stage, stage three the traditional stage, and stage four the realistic stage.[9,15] In the first stage man explained natural phenomena as magical, religious, or supernatural events. The physician was considered to be a god or priest. In the second stage knowledge was based partly on observation, but mainly on speculation. The doctor of this stage considered himself a philosopher. Two of the most well-known philosophers during this stage were Hippocrates and Aristotle: however, the most outstanding example was Claudius Galen (131 AD). Von Leden states that Galen was probably the most influential medical author of all time, as well as being the founder of laryngology and the godfather of phoniatrics and voice science. In the third stage all information was based on tradition or revelation, on the great authorities of the ancient world, and on the Fathers of the Church. Great healers of this stage include Christ, St. Luke, and St. Blaise. Those considered the greatest physicians and scientists of all time were Galen, Hippocrates, and Aristotle. During this stage there was a great anatomist named Mondino de Luzzi (1275-1327) of Cologne. However, Galen was still considered correct even if there was a discrepancy between his book and the live dissections by de Luzzi. In the fourth stage knowledge was based on actual observation, experimentation, and coordination. This stage was the beginning of medical science where physicians were expected to become proficient in both art and science. Anatomy professor, Leonardo da Vinci (1452-1510), must be given credit for being the pioneer of this era. He contributed new and important information to the anatomy, physiology, and pathology of the human voice.[15]

Von Leden further states that it must be noted at this point that early in the 18th century, Giovanni Battista Morgagni (1582-1771) was so influential in the field that he should be considered the second founder of laryngology. He clearly demonstrated that the larynx is the site of disease and that changes in function are related to pathologic changes.[15]

In the 19th century many important discoveries were made that helped to facilitate better understanding of the voice. The interior of a human larynx was observed for the first time, sound was described as arising from a series of puffs, the vibration of falsetto tones was examined, and the speech center of the brain was described. Two other major contributors include the outstanding physiologist Johannes Muller (1801-1858), who proclaimed the myoelastic theory of phonation in 1839, and Hermann von Helmholz (1821-1894), who pioneered the acoustics of sound.[15] One final important contributor to the field of laryngology and voice science, Spaniard Manuel García II (1805-1906), merits some discussion. However, before a discussion of García's contributions can ensue, it is necessary to give a brief account of some attempts at viewing the larynx prior to García.

From 1807 to 1829 there were actually a series of attempts at creating a device for laryngeal examination. Many medical professionals doubted the effective use of a mirror for examining the larynx even as late as 1832. Another citation of using a mirror to aid in laryngeal examination can be found in a book entitled *Practical Surgery* by Robert Liston in 1837.[4] Moore[16] states that one of the main problems of these investigations was insufficient light into the larynx for adequate viewing. Attempts at rectifying this problem were made by Adam Warden and by a Mr. Avery of London in 1844. These events bring us to the name that is most likely on the best known in the history of laryngoscopy: Manuel García II.

Singing teacher Manuel García II was the first to effectively use the laryngeal mirror for routine visualization of the larynx. Moore states that García "should be given credit for his original thinking" since he was most likely unaware of previous work in this area

(p. 267).[16] In 1854 García bought a dentist's mirror from the surgical instrument maker Charrière for 6 francs. This particular mirror had been dismissed as being inconsequential at the London exhibition in 1851. When he returned home, he placed the dental mirror against his uvula while holding another mirror in his hand onto which flashed a ray of sunlight. With these two mirrors and sunlight, he was able to observe his vocal folds in action. He wrote a description of what he saw and presented his paper titled "Physiological Observations of the Human Voice" to the Royal Society of London in 1855. As far as García was concerned, he had proven his theories and that the viewing of the vocal cords (vocal folds) with a laryngoscope (laryngeal mirror) ceased to be of any special use. His findings were initially received with indifference by the medical profession, and it was 2 years before the medical field realized the importance of the instrument.[8] García's contribution is evident not only in the general fields of laryngology and voice science, but also within a new subspecialization. The evolution of this new specialized field, arts medicine, can be traced to the era of Manuel García II.[4]

Arts Medicine Centers

Today, when a singer has a voice problem, it is advantageous to seek medical care from a voice care team at an Arts Medicine Center specializing in Professional Voice Care. As stated above, most Arts Medicine Centers are located in large metropolitan areas such as seen in Figure 3–2. The Thomas Jefferson University Hospital Arts Medicine Center, Philadelphia, Pa, was the third Arts Medicine Center in the nation to be established, with Northwestern and Cleveland Clinic being the first and second, respectively.[17] There were very few centers when Arts Medicine began but now more centers are springing up nationally as well as internationally. Log on to the Web site http://www.voicefoundation.org or contact the Voice Foundation to find an Arts Medicine Center nearest to you. On the Voice Foundation Web site, there is a membership listing and many of the leading voice care professionals are on this list. The Voice Foundation membership is composed of doctors, speech-language pathologists, singing voice specialists, voice scientists, acting voice specialists, and others from a variety of disciplines. The membership listing is accessible by region nationally (East, Midwest, South, and West) as well as internationally.[18]

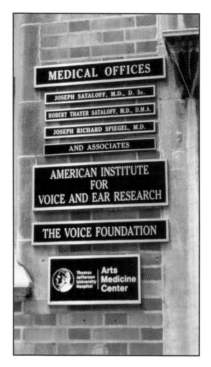

Figure 3–2. Thomas Jefferson University Hospital Arts Medicine Center, Philadelphia, Pennsylvania. Dr. Robert T. Sataloff, Director. This was the third center to be established in the nation.

Professional Voice Care Team

The Professional Voice Care Team is an interdisciplinary team composed of an otolaryngologist or laryngologist, a speech-language pathologist (SLP) or phoniatrist, a singing voice specialist (SVS), an acting voice specialist, a nurse and/or a physician's assistant, and consultant physicians in other specialties.[3] In addition, a voice scientist, stress manager/speaking coach, and a medical psychologist may be involved.

Definition of the Team Members. In a 2002 article in the *Journal of Singing*,[3] Heman-Ackah, Sataloff, and Hawkshaw define the team members as follows: (1) an otolaryngologist (ENT) is a physician/surgeon who practices all aspects of ear/nose/throat medicine whereas a laryngologist is a physician specializing in disorders of the larynx and voice and related problems as well, (2) a speech-language pathologist (SLP) is a certified, licensed healthcare professional with either a master's or Ph.D. degree, (3) a phoniatrist is a European voice care professional who is a physician that does not perform surgery but has also received training much like an American speech-language pathologist, and (4) a singing voice specialist (SVS) is a singing teacher with special training equipping him or her to practice in a medical environment with patients who have sustained vocal injury.

The role of the singing voice specialist in the team management of voice patients includes four main facets. The first is as a liaison between (1) patient and laryngologist, (2) patient and the voice scientist, (3) patient and speech-language pathologist, and (4) patient and the voice teacher. The second is as an educator. Education includes helping the patient understand the anatomy and physiology of phonation, what his/her diagnosis means for the current function of the singing voice, and what to expect vocally. This education will aid in reduction of the patient's anxiety level and help him/her cope emotionally. The third facet is as a trainer. A trainer helps the professional voice user to maximize the balance of the vocal system. The term trainer is synonymous with an athlete. If a professional athlete has a physical problem then he or she would most likely see a sports medicine specialist for therapy to mediate the problem. The singer is a vocal athlete. As there is no licensure for a singing voice specialist, legally the term therapist is not advocated. The fourth facet is as a problem solver. This facet will vary greatly depending on the patient's area of expertise. Additionally, there are elements of counseling that occur during a session.[19]

Protocol/Testing

The Professional Voice Care team will guide the singer through a progression of tests. The protocol consists of a medical diagnosis, objective measures, and a functional diagnosis of both the speaking and singing voice. Depending on the clinic, the medical diagnosis may come either before or after the objective measures. Once the singer has completed both the medical diagnosis and objective measures he or she will undergo a functional diagnosis.[20]

Subjective Testing. It is necessary for the otolaryngologist to collect an extensive historical background in order to adequately evaluate and diagnose the singer's vocal complaints.[4] After the physician has collected a thorough patient history, he/she must include an assessment of his/her general physical condition and a thorough ear, nose, and throat evaluation (Figure 3–3).

It should be noted that any maladies of almost any body system, not just conditions of the head and neck, may result in voice dysfunction. According to Sataloff, any patient with a voice complaint should at least be examined by indirect laryngoscopy.[4] There are many ENT's, who even today, feel that the exam is complete after viewing the vocal folds with use of the laryngeal mirror. However, in cases where further analysis is warranted, misdiagnoses may occur if the special procedure of strobovideolaryngoscopy (SVL) is not carried out. It has been documented in a study by Sataloff, Spiegel, and Hawkshaw, that a review of 1,876 clinical cases showed that SVL provides valuable information and alters diagnosis and/or treatment in approximately one-third of the patients for whom the procedure is indicated.[21] Currently, digital strobovideolaryngoscopy (SVL) is the standard of testing equipment (Figure 3–4).

Stroboscopy is the process of viewing the vocal folds by using either a rigid telescope (Figure 3–5) or flexible endoscope (Figure 3–6) which is attached to a flashing light source whose rate of flashing may be synchronized or desynchronized with the frequency of vocal fold motion or movement.[9]

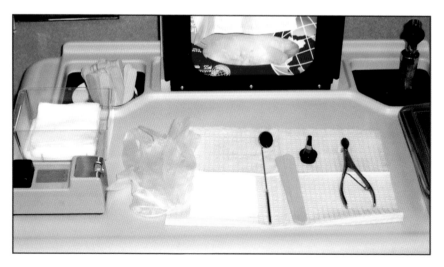

Figure 3–3. Setup for a thorough ear/nose/throat examination complete with the laryngeal mirror.

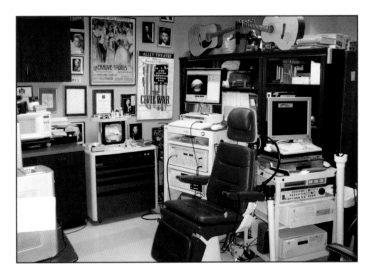

Figure 3-4. Texas Voice Center digital stroboscopy examination room setup. Dr. C. Richard Stasney, Director.

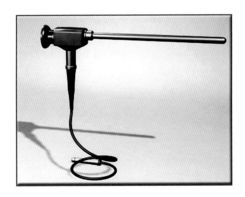

Figure 3-5. The rigid telescope instrument for viewing of the larynx.

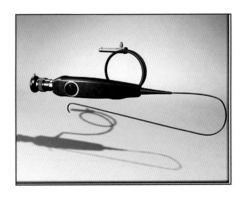

Figure 3-6. The flexible endoscope instrument for viewing of the larynx.

When viewing the vocal fold image with strobovideolaryngoscopy, it is important to know that right and left are switched due to being viewed through a camera lens. Furthermore, the size is magnified. It is possible to compare the exact size of the vocal folds to a dime, penny and quarter. Newborns have an average pitch (fundamental frequency = F_o) of 490 hertz which is perceived of as approximately B4 above middle C (C4). The mobile edges of the newborn vocal folds are about one-third to one-half the diameter of a dime. Before puberty, both sexes have a pitch that rests around 250 hertz (Hz) which is between B3 (just below middle C) and C4. Adult females drop to 200 Hz and their vocal fold length is around two-thirds the diameter of a penny. The adult male voice drops to approximately 110 Hz (basses are closer to 90 Hz and tenors around 115) and the mobile edges of the vocal folds are on average around two-thirds of the diameter of a quarter (Figure 3–7). Figure 3–8 shows the comparison of what is seen with strobovideo-laryngoscopy and the actual size of the female vocal folds.[6]

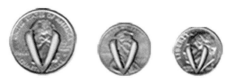

Figure 3–7. The approximate vocal fold sizes compared to a dime (child), penny (adult female), and quarter (adult male).

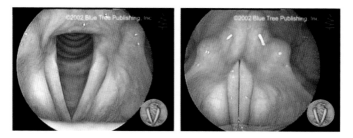

Figure 3–8. An examination of the adult female vocal folds with the procedure of digital stroboscopy viewed in open and closed position. In the right-hand corner notice the comparison of the approximate actual size as compared to the magnified view of stroboscopy.

Strobovideolaryngoscopy is a subjective test. A subjective assessment is an evaluation based on observation, perception, and opinion, rather than independently reproducible quantifiable measures.[4] A common analogy would be that of a doctor evaluating a CT scan or x-ray. Because this is a picture (like stroboscopy—internally viewing the vocal folds), the diagnosis is only as good as the knowledge of the one making the diagnosis. The equipment can be exemplary but if the doctor making the evaluation is not well versed in the singer's condition, then a misdiagnosis may occur. During the medical diagnosis, it is indispensable for the singer to be examined with both the rigid telescope and the flexible endoscope. Both tests give vital information that will be used by the voice care team for diagnoses and treatment. A rigid laryngeal telescope via stroboscopy allows for the best evaluation of the vibratory parameters of voice whereas flexible endoscopy allows for best evaluation of the singer's dynamic use of voice (e.g. singing, speaking, functional tasks). Often the laryngologist will only offer a rigid stroboscopic examination; however, it is essential for the singing voice specialist to see functionally what a singer is doing when performing. If the singer sings more than one style, it is necessary for him/her to sing a few lines of each style. This information will aid in both functional analysis and treatment plan development.

Objective Testing. An objective assessment primarily involves instrumentation which has quantifiable (scientific) data that has been collected over years of research such as pulmonary function testing where a patient will be compared to others of the same age, weight, sex, height, and race. Norms have also been established for acoustic and phonatory measures. Common objective assessment includes acoustic, phonatory, and respiratory measures.

Although x-rays and CT-scans do exist, the preferred noninvasive assessment of sound is by use of acoustic measures. There are a variety of systems available but one of the most compact and powerful systems is the the Kay/Pentax Computerized Speech Lab (CSL)[22] which has a variety of measurement tools. Ideally, we will reach Dr. Sataloff's vision of standardizing objective measures such that we will have one instrument, like the audiometer, to acoustically view the voice.[4] It is interesting to note that Dr. Gould (1987) outlined the idea of a voice analysis network in which laboratories could tie into a central computer. Today, we are now closer than ever before to reaching Sataloff's ideal for acoustic analysis. Kay/Pentax, the manufacturers of the DSP Sona-Graph, are now producing the Computer Speech Lab (CSL) with many options including the Visi-Pitch IV (VPIV), Sona-Match (SNM), and the Multi-Dimensional Voice Program (MDVP) but to name a few (Figures 3-9A and 3-9B).[22]

Common phonatory measures include: (1) Speaking Fundamental Frequency, (2) Physiologic Frequency Range of Phonation (PFRP) —measurement of the lowest tone to the highest tone physiologically, and (3) Musical Frequency Range of Phonation (MFRP)—measurement of the lowest tone to the highest tone musically. Both the lower and the higher limits must be held for 1 to 2 seconds and (4) s/z ratio which measures vocal fold closure completeness. Some clinics also add maximum phonation time (MPT) which is the measurement of the maximum time that a subject phonates on and both spoken and sung production of the vowels /ɑ/, /i/ and /u/. MPT is measured using a hand-held stopwatch, accurate to 1/100 of a second.[9]

The last group of objective tests includes respiratory measures and glottal efficiency assessment. Pulmonary function tests are measurements which help to determine the ability of the lungs and abdomen to support speech and singing. Although a variety of instruments are available for measuring respiratory function, the spirometer is commonly used in the Arts Medicine Voice Laboratory. The pulmonary function test (PFT) measures used clinically in the voice lab include (1) FVC—forced vital capacity—the total amount of air a subject can expel during the entire exhalation process, (2) FEV 1.0—forced expiratory volume—the amount of air expelled during the first second of exhalation and (3) FEF 25-75%—forced expiratory flow in the 25 to 75% range—the amount of air expelled during the middle of the exhalation (Figure 3-10). Last, Mean Flow Rate (MFR) is a measurement of laryngeal airflow during phonation on the vowel /ɑ/ to examine glottal efficiency.[9]

Functional Diagnoses. The next evaluation step for the voice professional is a functional evaluation by either the speech-language pathologist (SLP) or the singing voice specialist (SVS). The functional evaluation will determine what treatment plan is necessary for remediation of the vocal disorder.

The speaking voice evaluation by the speech-language pathologist can be divided into four parts: (1) case history, (2) examination, (3) assessment, and (4) recommendations. Once the case history has been collected, the speech-language pathologist subjectively evaluates

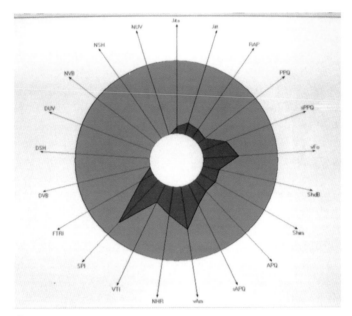

A

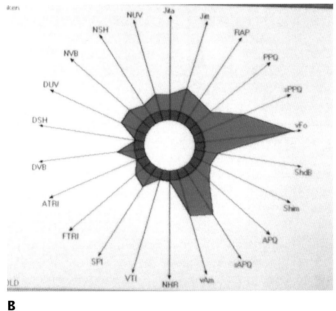

B

Figure 3-9. **A.** A normal acoustic voiceprint using the Kay Elemetrics MDVP. **B.** A disordered acoustic voiceprint using the Kay Elemetrics MDVP.

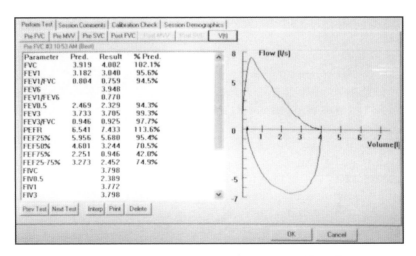

Figure 3–10. Pulmonary Function Test (PFT) flow loop.

the singer's speaking voice production. The SLP listens to functional behaviors of (1) frequency (pitch), (2) intensity (loudness), timing rate of speech), (3) timing (rate of speech), and (4) quality (roughness, hoarseness, etc.).[23] Other important things evaluated are (1) sites of muscular tension, (2) the oral/facial mechanism, and (3) the number of harsh glottal attacks counted during a standard reading task. The therapist will use trial therapy during the examination to determine what therapy will be useful. After the evaluation, recommendations are made concerning if therapy is needed and any therapy goals are defined.[4]

The next evaluation step for the professional voice user is the singing voice evaluation. Although a history has been obtained by the otolaryngologist and speech-language pathologist, the singer, either consciously or unconsciously, may have omitted important pertinent information. Singers are often more comfortable acknowledging and expressing how devastated they are by their situation to the singing voice specialist (SVS). The SVS may be the first member of the team to recognize the influence of psychological factors which may impair response to medical and surgical therapy.[19] Therefore, history is the first important item during the initial evaluation. After discussing the singer's history and voice use, a subjective evaluation of the singer's vocal system characteristics is obtained while he or she sings a five-note ascending/descending scale on /a/ up and down by half steps.

These characteristics are logged onto a checklist and then discussed with the singer. The singer is then asked to sing a selection from something in his/her style(s) of music. During this time the SVS will look for misalignment of the "system's balance."[24] The vocal system must be evaluated before therapy can ensue. Specific points of assessment include: (1) Stance/posture, (2) breathing and support, (3) placement, (4) quality of voice, (5) current range, and (6) tension points. Some terms which are commonly used in the voice world are actually misnomers—such as placement. This term makes it sound like the voice is an object to be held and put somewhere. But this debate is for another time! The training begins once the evaluation and discussion have been completed. The exercises are chosen based on the professional discipline/genre, situation, and health of each individual singer.

General Body Health

Medical Disclaimer

One may wonder why there is a discussion of general body health issues prior to discussion of specific vocal health issues. Remember that this is pertinent as the singing voice is composed of the body/mind/spirit. Therefore, when you medically treat the physical body it has the potential to affect the voice. The following recommendations of general health are primarily from the CD-ROM Vocal Health[6] as well as information disseminated by the Texas Voice Center; C. Richard Stasney, M.D., Director.[25] It is not the intent of this segment to offer a complete guide for self-care of the singing voice. Neither is it the intent of this segment to offer complete medical information about care of all the various ailments. Rather, this segment attempts to emphasize the high points of vocal health and the most important common afflictions that affect singers.[6] It is important for singers to be under the care of a laryngologist who specializes in professional voice care and to consult their physician about pertinent health issues.

It is necessary to discuss general body health issues prior to discussing specific vocal health issues as the body is the vocal instrument. Issues to be considered are: (1) Life Health Issues, (2) Drying Agents, (3) Medications, and (4) Acid Reflux.

Life Health Issues: Hydration, Balanced Diet, Rest, and Exercise

Hydration. Normal Vocal Fold Requirements. Normal healthy vocal folds require a thin layer of mucus to vibrate efficiently. The thin layer of mucous helps lubricate the vocal folds in a manner similar to oil in a car engine. Much like a car engine without oil, vocal folds without lubrication do not operate properly and can be damaged. Therefore, vocal folds must have this lubrication to vibrate well. To maintain lubrication of the vocal folds, the entire body must have adequate hydration. Adequate hydration can be achieved by drinking plenty of water every day. Some clinics recommend as much as 8 to 10 glasses of water a day. Drinking water several hours before prolonged voice use will give the body enough time to absorb the fluids so that the vocal folds vibrate with ease.[6]

One of the most common causes of voice problems is speaking/ singing with dry vocal folds (vocal cords). If the body does not have enough fluids to be hydrated properly, the vocal folds become dry and function poorly. If you have *few* demands on the voice, you may never experience vocal problems due to dry vocal folds. However, this is rarely the case with voice users. Singers tend to have very high demands on the voice and singing with dehydrated vocal folds frequently results in vocal problems such as a hoarse voice, voice breaks, loss of volume or pitch range, vocal fatigue, and loss of voice. If a physician looks at your vocal folds with a mirror or other more sophisticated equipment and sees dryness of the vocal folds (thick mucus), they will refer to this condition as *laryngitis sicca*. Although this is one of the most frequent causes of vocal problems, it is also one of the easiest to cure.[6]

Balanced Diet. In this age of fast food and prepared meals, it is often difficult to eat healthily. Many people eat in their cars and on the run. It is important to remember that the food you eat is much like gas for a car. Dr. Robert J. Moore III[26] describes how food affects our bodies very clearly. He states that the type, amounts and combinations of the macronutrients (carbohydrates, protein, and fat) that we eat are the fuel for our body and that indeed we really are what we eat (p. 13). We need to treat ourselves with care if we want to endure. Would you put leaded gas or diesel fuel in a Jaguar? Probably not, and yet we often mistreat our physical bodies and health by the fuel that we consume.

Rest. There are many things in the body that are rejuvenated during sleep. When tired, there is the inclination to be less mentally sharp. This can cause one to eat more. One can also feel dehydrated from lack of sleep. Furthermore, lack of sleep can cause physical fatigue and make one more prone to accidents.[27] Singers need to be mentally and physically prepared for the game!

Exercise. Many people think that exercise implies getting a membership at a local gymnasium. This is definitely an excellent option if you wish to do so. However, there are ways to put exercise into your daily routine. For instance, when you go to the store, do not drive around until the parking spot nearest the door is available. Park farther away and walk to the door. Also, if you need to go up a few flights in a building, it would be of benefit to take the stairs instead of going up the elevator. Another idea would be to walk around in your neighborhood, park, parking lot of a local church, or mall. I often like to do more than one thing at a time so I read articles while I am on my treadmill or stationary bicycle.

A final note needs to be mentioned in regard to balanced diet, rest, and exercise. These life health issues are incredibly important in reducing the stress factor in life. More and more the medical field is finding that stress can be a major factor in many diseases. Therefore, it behooves all to work stress relief into the daily life balance. It is important to find what works for each individual in regard to stress release.

Drying Agents/Factors

There are causes for dehydration other than not drinking enough water. Common drying agents/factors include (1) Caffeine, (2) Alcohol, (3) Diuretics, (4) Medications, and (5) Environmental effects.

Caffeine/Alcohol/Diuretics. Caffeinated drinks such as coffee, tea and most soft drinks tend to dehydrate because they cause the body to remove fluids from the tissue (act like a diuretic). This does not mean that you can't have your café mocha or your early morning "eye opener." The important point is to balance the caffeine by increasing the amount of water you drink. People often ask if drinking other liquids such as fruit juices or decaffeinated coffee/tea is as effective as drinking water. Although these choices are better than caffeinated drinks, water is clearly the best choice for the voice. Alcohol, like caffeine, pulls water out of your system and depletes the vocal folds of necessary lubrication. Alcohol also has the added factor of being acidic which can aggravate any problems with reflux (to be discussed).[6] Another effect of caffeine is found through the use of over-the-counter diuretics. Diuretics are often used to deplete excess water.[28]

Medications. Along with the antihistamines (discussed below), there are other medications that may cause dehydration and dryness of the vocal folds. Many antidepressants can also have a drying effect on the vocal folds. If the benefit of these medications exceeds the risk of dryness, they must be used, but the patient should be aware of this side effect.[6] Be sure to consult your physician (CYP) in regard to finding the best choice of medications for you, the singer.

Effects of Environment. Dry environments deplete the body of needed water, which can affect the voice. These symptoms are usually worse during winter months. This includes the outside climate and inside environment. Air conditioning and heaters reduce the amount of moisture in the air. Fans (especially those directed at the face) dry you out by evaporating body moisture. The important issue is to increase the amount of water you drink when in a dry environment. An excellent remedy for a dry voice is to use a humidifier while you sleep.[6] Facial steamers, which provide direct mouth to moisture, may also be of benefit.

Effects of Medications

It is highly recommended that one read the information from the pharmacist in regard to the active ingredients and the effect of the ingredients on the body. This should hold true for the use of all medications. When in doubt, ask your pharmacist directly or consult your physician (CYP).

Antihistamines. Antihistamines and decongestants are sometimes prescribed to treat allergy, cold, or flu symptoms and are present in many over-the-counter cold medications. Be careful about using antihistamines (and even decongestants) because they tend to cause dryness of the vocal folds. Inhalers used for asthma can also cause dryness and irritation of the larynx.[6,25] There may be other medications or treatments that can relieve the symptoms without the drying side effects of antihistamines or inhalers (CYP).

Analgesics. Aspirin products and nonsteroidal anti-inflammatory drugs (ibuprofen) should be used with caution as they cause platelet dysfunction and this may predispose to bleeding. Tylenol (McNeil Consumer Products) is the best substitute for pain relief for the singer.[25]

Mucolytic Agents. Most people experience thick mucus in the nose, throat, or sinuses due to colds or chronic sinus or nasal problems. A common error is to take drying medications to alleviate the feeling of thick mucous. This *worsens* the problem by increasing the thickness of the mucous. A better remedy is to use a mucous thinning agent like guaifenesin to help liquefy the mucous. Mucolytic agents need to be taken with a lot of water daily to be effective. Another remedy that can work wonders is to use a humidifier while sleeping to add moisture to loosen up the mucous.[6,25]

Progesterone. Question the use of progesterone-dominant birth control pills. They may cause virilization of the female larynx and a loss in the upper vocal range. However, there may be no other alternative for your individual situation, so consult your gynecologist.[25]

Steroids. Steroids should be used with care and caution. If there is swelling it is important to discover what the underlying cause or problem is. Steroids are anti-inflammatory agents and are potentially helpful in managing acute inflammatory laryngitis. However, singers must be careful not to abuse steroids [28] (CYP).

Acid Reflux

What Is Reflux? When we eat something, the food reaches the stomach by traveling down a muscular tube called the esophagus. Once food reaches the stomach, the stomach adds acid and pepsin (a digestive enzyme) so that the food can be digested. The esophagus has two areas that act like sphincters (bands of muscle fibers that close off the tube) that help keep the contents of the stomach where they belong. One sphincter area is at the bottom of the esophagus (where the stomach and esophagus meet) and is called the lower esophageal sphincter or LES. Another sphincter area is at the top of the esophagus (where the esophagus and throat meet) and is called the upper esophageal sphincter or UES. The term reflux means "a backward or return flow," and usually refers to the backward flow of stomach contents up through the sphincters and into the esophagus or throat. There are two common types of reflux. One is GERD and the other is LPRD.[6,25]

Some people have an abnormal amount of reflux of stomach acid up through the lower sphincter and into the esophagus. This is referred to as GERD or Gastro-Esophageal Reflux Disease. If the reflux makes it all the way up through the upper sphincter and into the back of the throat, it is called LPRD or Laryngo- Pharyngeal Reflux Disease. The structures in the throat (pharynx, larynx) and lungs are much more sensitive to stomach acid so smaller amounts of reflux into these areas can result in more damage.[6,25]

Serious Reflux Can Occur Without Heartburn. People often assume that because they feel no heartburn then they do not have reflux. This is one of the main reasons that reflux is often misdiagnosed. The fact is that very few people with LPRD ever experience significant heartburn. Heartburn occurs when the tissue in the esophagus becomes irritated. Most of the reflux events that can damage the throat happen without the patient ever knowing that they are occurring. If you question that you may have reflux, a knowledgeable Laryngologist (Ear, Nose, and Throat or Otolaryngologist) can diagnose reflux-related voice problems. It is important to note that reflux can mimic other conditions such as asthma, postnasal drip, and sinus problems.[6]

Reflux Causes and Treatments. Just as symptoms differ from person to person, it must be understood that the combination of causes of reflux are unique to the person experiencing it. Some of the causes can be stress, types of food, amount of food at mealtimes, eating late at night, body weight, tight clothing, and smoking.[6] Sometimes monitoring stress, foods, body weight, and clothing is not enough. In the event that another course of treatment is warranted there are several over-the-counter remedies available as well as prescription and holistic approaches. There are excellent books to consult such as *Professional Voice: The Science and Art of Clinical Care* by Robert T. Sataloff and *The Performer's Voice* by Benninger and Murray. If you are a singer it is also possible to have singing induced reflux. Every time that you use good breath support you push against the lower esophageal sphincter. If you suspect that you have reflux related voice problems, your physician can help determine which treatment and level of medication would be best for you.

Traveling Concerns

It is important to be prepared when traveling as a singer. It is smart to have a traveling assortment of items that you routinely pack to aid in general body/vocal health. The travel pack suggestions include all prescription medications along with nose, throat, and body items. Review the suggestions below:

- Prescription Medications
- Nose
  - Saline Spray
  - Over-the-counter (OTC) Nasalcrom
    - Buffers against new allergens
- Throat
  - Entertainers Secret (1-800-308-7452)
    - Safe hydrating throat spray
  - Throat Coat Tea
    - "Traditional Medicinal" brand tea
  - Nonmenthol throat lozenges
- Body
  - Mucinex
    - Over-the-counter mucus thinning agent
  - Tylenol
  - Tums, Gaviscon
    - Over-the-counter antacids

Along with the travel pack suggestions there are a few other issues to consider. The pressurized air that is supplied on airplanes will tend to have a serious drying effect on your voice. If you are asked to fly to a singing engagement, start drinking water several hours prior to the flight and continue throughout the flight.[25]

Last, it is wise to limit voice use while on a plane; especially if one has to rehearse or perform shortly after landing. A beneficial treatment when arriving is to steam the body for rehydration. This can be done by showering, soaking in a steamy tub, or by turning on the hot water in the sink, or putting a towel over your head and breathing in the steam. Of course, a facial steamer may also be used.

Studio Concerns

There are also issues to be prepared for when studio recording. Studio concerns include physical comfort, vocal technique, and studio technique issues. In regard to physical comfort it is important to be prepared to hydrate yourself with water (not cold), tea such as "throat coat" tea mentioned above, and if desired, "Entertainer's Secret" throat spray. It will be important to let the recording engineer or producer know how much time you will be able to sing before you need to have some vocal rest. Another physical comfort issue is being prepared for warmer/cooler temperatures in the studio. It is smart to layer what you are wearing (i.e., t-shirt, sweatshirt, etc.). A final issue of concern is what to eat when recording. It is smart to be aware of and avoid anything that may cause reflux to occur such as highly spiced or fatty foods.

If you are paying by the hour for a project, it is wise to arrive musically and vocally prepared at the studio. Many singers like to arrive early to get physically comfortable in the space as well as spend time with body/voice preparation (warm-up). If you are paying a lump sum for the project, the singer often feels a bit less pressure to quickly perform and is able to experiment with style and interpretation. However, this does not mean to be vocally ill-prepared as no engineer/producer likes to waste time.

Studio technique issues include learning what makes you comfortable when recording. One issue is to decide if you prefer to have both headphones on while singing to the instrumental tracks or if you prefer to have only one headphone on. It is also important to let your engineer/producer know if the levels of the music track and vocals that you are hearing through the headphone(s) are acceptable. If it is too loud then the singer will pull back in volume and if it is too soft the singer will most likely oversing.[29] Another issue is becoming comfortable with use of a microphone. The setting and placement of the microphone is important as well as the choice of microphone (Figures 3–11A and 3–11B).

It is also of interest to note that advances in technology now allow a singer to record a voice track to a prepared music track in one studio and then send the wave files to a producer in another studio to do the final mix. This can happen from place to place via the Internet (Figures 3–12A, 3–12B, and 3–12C).

It can be unsettling to hear your own voice the first few times when recording. Often singers get caught in the trap of criticizing and critiquing the sound and then begin to compensate and control the voice by holding at the larynx (i.e., with neck muscles or glottal tension) to improve the sound. There is also a temptation to oversing. Remember that this kind of singing will eventually cause problems. Refer to Chapters 1 and 2 to review how sound is produced and how to play your instrument. It is not necessary to push the voice when recording. The microphone simply records what you are doing and a good engineer/producer will know what to do to maximize your performance (Figures 3–13A and 3–13B).

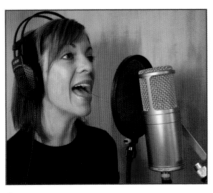 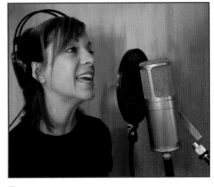

A   **B**

Figure 3–11. **A.** Microphone positioning in a professional studio setting with both ears covered by headset. **B.** Microphone positioning in a professional studio setting with one ear covered by headset.

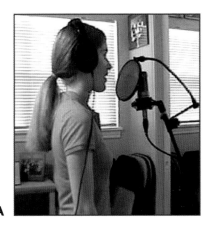

A

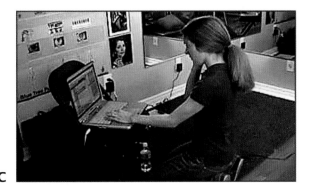

B

C

Figure 3-12. **A.** Traveling studio setup. **B.** A professional music program on a laptop for collecting wave files of music. **C.** Singer/ songwriter checking to see if the capture of the take was to her liking.

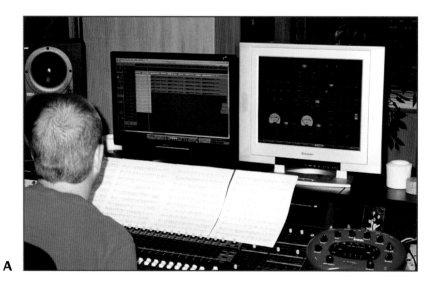

A

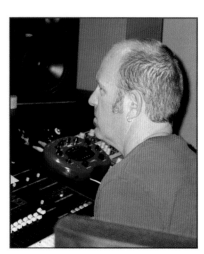

B

Figure 3-13.
A. Professional music studio, Coach Beiden Music. **B.** Doug Beiden, producer, Coach Beiden Music.

Voice Care

As a singer your body is your instrument. Therefore, care of the singing voice includes all of the general health information discussed as well as your speaking voice habits and technique. General voice care techniques are discussed along with speaking voice, and singing voice care is presented.

General Voice Care: Sound Production

It is important to remember that we only have one larynx which is responsible for many tasks. These tasks include: (1) speaking, (2) singing, (3) yelling, (4) screaming, (5) coughing, (6) throat clearing, and (7) crying. Remember that the larynx is also the passage for the airway.

General Voice Care Techniques. Important voice care techniques include ways that we limit voice use as well as behaviors to avoid. In order to have vocal longevity and minimize vocal damage, it is smart to (1) limit the use of the voice in high noise environments, (2) limit the amount of general voice use before a performance, and (3) think "voice conservation." Self-destructive behaviors to avoid include: (1) smoking, (2) harsh throat clearing, (3) screaming, (4) talking above background noise, (5) yelling and screaming at sporting events, and (6) attention-getting (yelling and shouting from room to room or across a long distance). Other non-work-related issues of concern that can also affect healthy voice production include: (1) social obligations, (2) civic or religious committees or organizations, (3) late night eating, (4) prior vocal problems, (5) medical history, and (6) phone time at home. It would be of further benefit to know if the singer has had any previous singing voice lessons or any speaking voice training.

Vocal Health

Vocal health for speaking and singing includes all of the general body health issues discussed above as well as the general voice care techniques. Along with the above issues is the question of what percentage during the day is the voice "on" and what percentage of the day is the voice "off" or resting.

It is important to monitor in what way(s) and how much the voice is being used. Ways include what activity as well as technique. Singing voice activities include things such as (1) enjoyment along with the radio/CD, (2) choral ensembles, (3) solo singing, (4) musical theatre productions, and (5) recording. Speaking voice activities include (1) conversation—live and on the phone (2) theatre productions, as well as (3) instruction and discipline if one has children or teaches religious or community classes. A singer thinks about the need for having a technique for singing but often does not think technically about how they speak. Healthy vocal technique for sound production, whether speaking or singing, includes (1) pitch, (2) resonance, (3) air-flow management—breath control/support, (4) rate of speed, and (5) volume level.

Common Disorders

If singers are not mindful of taking care of their voices with general body health and vocal health, potential problems may occur. Common disorders include functional maladies such as muscular tension dysphonia (MTD), also known as hyperfunction, as well as common medical pathologies such as (1) reflux, (2) nodules, (3) polyp, and (4) hemorrhage. It would be wise to review what normal vocal folds look like at this point in order to be able to compare them with a disordered larynx (Figure 3–14).

Functional. Muscle tension dysphonia (MTD), also known as hyper-function, is actually a very common vocal condition where there is excessive muscular activity involved in the larynx. This functional condition may be associated as a compensational behavior with a medical pathology or it may exist as a singular diagnosis. When a singer or speaker has this condition, the vocal folds and the area around the vocal folds squeeze together too tightly. Typically the singer or speaker is completely unaware that this is occurring. There are two common configurations of MTD. One is by using anterior/posterior compression (front to back squeezing) as seen in Figure 3–15A and the other is called medial/lateral constriction (both sides squeezing

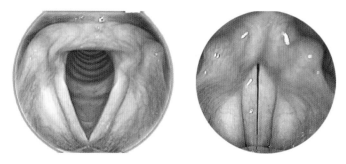

Figure 3–14. Open and closed views of normal vocal folds.

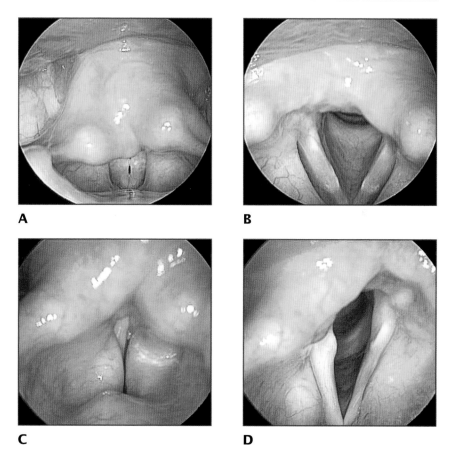

Figure 3-15. **A.** Anterior/posterior muscle tension dysphonia (MTD) closed view. **B.** AP MTD open view. **C.** Medial/lateral muscle tension dysphonia (MTD) closed view. **D.** ML MTD open view.

toward the center) where the false vocal folds are squeezed toward the midline or center as seen in Figure 3-15C. Notice that for both configuration even the open views have evidence of muscular over-work (Figures 3-15B and 3-15D). Potential signs that can be evidence of MTD includes (1) vocal fatigue/tiredness, (2) loss of "focus" of tones, (3) voice "cuts out," (4) loss of notes in the upper register, (5) reduction of vocal flexibility, (6) frequent episodes of voice loss, (7) tightness in the throat, (8) pain or soreness in the muscles of the neck surrounding the larynx, (9) change in voice quality, (10) pressed or stressed sound, and (11) persistently hoarse/breathy voice. It is imperative that a singer see his/her laryngologist who specializes in professional voice care if any of these symptoms persist. This is important because a general ENT who does not routinely see professional voices may conclude that nothing is wrong as this is a muscular problem with often no visible pathology present.[30] After the diagnosis by the Laryngologist, the singer will need to see a SLP and/or SVS who specialize(s) in behavioral management to remediate the functional problem.

Medical. As stated earlier, reflux is a very common problem for singers. The very nature of the technique for singing can result in a type of reflux called "singing induced reflux." Use of excellent airflow management (breath support/control) causes the abdomen to push against the lower esophageal sphincter which may in turn cause the LES to loosen and cause reflux to occur. The appearance of reflux can be varied and many. Sometimes it occurs alone and sometimes it occurs with pathology such as a polyp, granuloma or ulcer. The three examples of reflux shown are examples of reflux without an associated pathology (Figures 3–16A through 3–16C). Common medical symptoms of reflux include hoarseness, chronic cough, frequent throat clearing, pain or sensation in the throat, feeling of a lump in the throat, bad/bitter taste in the mouth, asthmalike symptoms, referred ear pain, and postnasal drip. Singing symptoms include extended warm-up time, difficulty with high notes, and a feeling like there is a veil or covering over the voice that you need to punch or push through. Strong signs seen by the doctor that you may have reflux include red/irritated arytenoids, red/irritated larynx, and swelling of the vocal folds.[6] If the reflux event occurs when the vocal folds are apart then the trachea will most likely be splashed with acid as well. This will be seen as a red/irritated trachea.

Another common singing ailment is bilateral vocal folds nodules. Nodules used to be the term for any growth seen on the vocal folds. Now the term "nodules" is reserved for bilateral lesions on the vocal folds[31] that create an hourglass configuration upon the closed vocal fold cycle. They are benign (noncancerous) growths on the surface of the vocal folds generally caused by chronic vocal abuse and occur most commonly in children and women (Figure 3–17). Nodules are often called "vocal fold calluses" because they are caused by a behavior much like the calluses on the feet caused by shoes that are too tight;

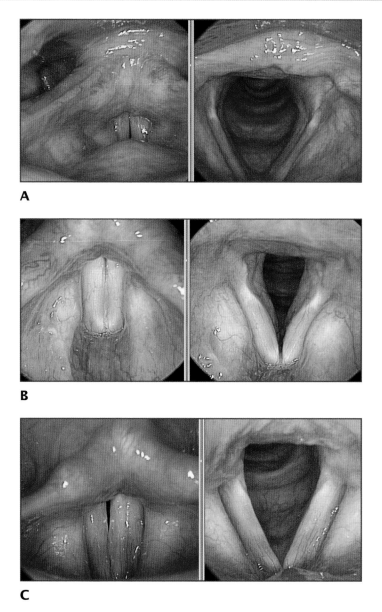

A

B

C

***Figure 3–16.* A, B**, and **C**. Vocal folds with reflux.

they result from repetitive irritation.[32] The abusive behavior must stop and the technique must be retrained for the pathology to resolve. If surgery is recommended without retraining, the singer

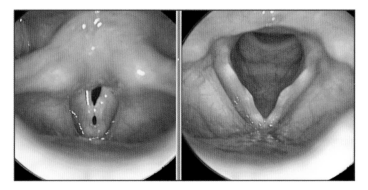

Figure 3-17. Vocal fold nodules.

should consult with another specialist. Also if vocal fold stripping is recommended—run! This is an antiquated surgical technique which is not in use by highly trained surgeons anymore.

The term "polyp," like reflux, may also have a variety of appearances and differ in location and type. A polyp may occur when one overuses the voice when the vocal folds are irritated or inflamed such as with an acute respiratory illness. Common types include (1) Angiomatous-blood filled, (2) Gelatinous, and (3) Fibrous polyps. They are connected to the vocal fold by a base or by a stem/stalk. They are benign (noncancerous) and usually unilateral (on one side). The term polyp is a descriptive term rather than a histologic (tissue) diagnosis. In Figure 3-18 in the closed vocal fold view the polyp has actually moved so that it rests on top of the right vocal fold which allows for better contact of both vocal folds together than if the polyp stayed at the vocal fold level.[28,32]

A reason to cancel a concert and to close the lips, other than post vocal fold surgery, is a vocal fold hemorrhage. A vocal hemorrhage is when a blood vessel bursts and bleeds into the vocal folds. It is absolutely critical to go on voice rest, typically for one to two weeks, in order for the hemorrhage to resolve so that no permanent vocal damage occurs (e.g., scar) (Figure 3-19).

It is important to note that most benign (noncancerous) vocal fold disorders as mentioned above, are associated with cumulative phonotrauma (abusive vf behavior) and repeated occurrences of hoarseness are not necessary or good. Vocal fold problems are rarely sudden (except vocal fold hemorrhage) but instead have a gradual onset.

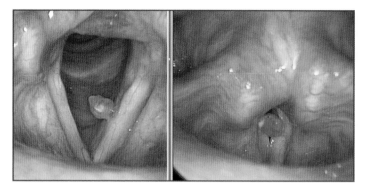

Figure 3–18. Left vocal fold polyp.

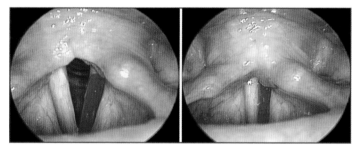

Figure 3–19. Left vocal fold hemorrhage.

Conclusion

It is essential for vocal health and longevity of voice use to apply the general body and vocal health advice presented here. Part of this application includes in what way(s) and how much the voice is used. It is also imperative to remember that there is efficient, healthy technique that is necessary for the speaking voice as well as the singing voice. As we only have one instrument, what we do when we are not singing will directly affect what we do when we sing; both good and bad. In addition, we speak more than we sing.

We live in an age where it is advisable as well as possible to see a Laryngologist who specializes in professional voice care within the field of Arts Medicine. There have been many advances in voice science and medicine since García's first view of the vocal folds and the

Helmholz resonator. Current technology not only has made it possible to view the vocal folds but also allows objective acoustical analysis of singing and speaking. Today there are numerous workshops and symposia which deal with the scientific aspects of voice function and voice care. Scientifically oriented articles are also found in the *National Association of Teachers of Singing (NATS) Journal.* The *Journal of Voice* (JOV), which began publication in 1987, is specifically devoted to scientific aspects of the voice. Books of note include: (1) *Professional Voice: The Science and Art of Clinical Care* by Sataloff, (2) *Textbook of Performing Arts Medicine* by Sataloff, Brandfonbrener, and Lederman, (3) *Vocal Arts Medicine: The Care and Prevention of Professional Voice Disorders* by Benninger, Jacobson, and Johnson, and (4) *The Performer's Voice* by Benninger and Murry (refer to the suggested reading list at the end of this chapter for more titles). Educational CD-ROMs available by Blue Tree Publishing include titles such as: (1) Vocal Health, (2) Vocal Parts, (3) Respiration, and many others about pathologies, and so forth. It is currently not possible to receive a degree in arts medicine although the field has been in practice since 1987. A degree plan for a doctorate in arts medicine has been proposed but not yet approved.[33] A master's degree plan has also been proposed for preparing the singing voice specialist.[19] Arts medicine is a cross-disciplinary degree with no precedent. Acceptance is proving challenging but the undertaking continues.

Acknowledgments. The author thanks Melina Gonzalez, Dr. Robert T. Sataloff, Brenda Beiden, Becky Simon, and Doug Beiden for permission for figures in order: 3–1, 3–2, 3–11A and 3–12B, 3–12A through 3–12C and 3–13A and 3–13B.

The author thanks Dr. C. Richard Stasney (Texas Voice Center) for allowing the author to photograph the Texas Voice Center and for pictures for Figures 3–3, 3–4, 3–9A and 3–9B, 3–10, 3–14, 3–15A through 3–15D, 3–16A through 3–16C, 3–17, 3–18, and 3–19.

The author thanks Robert O'Brien (Blue Tree Publishing) for permission to use Figures 3–5, 3–6, 3–7, 3–8, and 3–14.

The author thanks *Journal of Voice* for permission to publish material from the article "Preparing the singing voice specialist revisited."

The author thanks *Texas Sings!* for republication of material from several journal articles.

References

1. Sataloff RT, Brandfonbrener AG, Lederman RJ, eds. *Textbook of Performing Arts Medicine*. New York, NY: Raven Press; 1991.
2. Heman-Ackah YD, Sataloff RT, Hawkshaw MJ. Who takes care of Voice Problems? A guide to voice care providers. *NATS Journal of Singing*. 2002;November/December:139-146.
3. Sataloff RT. Professional singers: the science and art of clinical care. *American Journal of Otolaryngology*. 1981;2(3):251-266.
4. Sataloff RT. *Professional Voice: The Science and Art of Clinical Care*. New York, NY: Raven Press; 1991.
5. Webster N, McKechnie J. *Webster's New Twentieth Century Dictionary Unabridged*. New York, NY: Simon and Schuster; 1983.
6. Garrett JD, Radionoff SL, Rodriguez M, Stasney CR. *Vocal Health*. Lynnewood, Wash: Blue Tree Publishing; 2003.
7. Coffin B. *Historical Vocal Pedagogy Classics*. Metuchen, NJ: Scarecrow Press; 1989.
8. MacKinlay RM. *García: The Centenarian and His Times*. New York, NY: Da Capo Press; 1908.
9. Radionoff SL. *Objective Measures of Vocal Production During the Course of Singing Study*. Doctoral dissertation. Michigan: Michigan State University; 1996. Available from: ProQuest Digital Dissertations. Retrieved September 8, 2007, Publication Number: AAT 9631333.
10. Miller R. *English, French, German and Italian Techniques of Singing: A Study in National Tonal Preferences and How They Relate to Functional Efficiency*. Metuchen, NJ: Scarecrow Press; 1977.
11. Reid C. *Bel Canto Principles and Practices*. New York, NY: The Joseph Patelson Music House; 1978.
12. Miller R. The Singing teacher in the age of voice science. In: Sataloff RT, ed. *Professional Voice: The Science and Art of Clinical Care*. New York, NY: Raven Press; 1991:375-380.
13. *Musical Courier*. New Publications in Review; microfilm. August 1951; 28.
14. García M II. *A Complete Treatise on the Art of Singing: Part 1*. New York, NY: Da Capo Press; 1984 (editions of 1841 and 1872 edited by Donald V. Paschke).
15. Von Leden H. The cultural history of the larynx and voice. In: Gould WJ, Sataloff RT, Spiegel JR, eds. *Voice Surgery*. St. Louis, Mo: Mosby; 1993.
16. Moore P. A Short history of laryngeal investigation. *Journal of Voice*. 1991;5(3):266-281.
17. Sataloff RT. Personal communication, June 20, 2007.

18. The Voice Foundation. Retrieved June 8, 2007 from http://www.voice foundation.org.

19. Radionoff SL. Preparing the singing voice specialist revisited. *Journal of Voice*, 2004;18:513–521.

20. Radionoff SL. *The Role of the Singing Voice Specialist in Team Management of Voice Care.* Paper presented at: 4th International Care of the Professional and Occupational Voice Symposium, Canadian Voice Care Foundation; May 4, 1999; Banff, Alberta, Canada.

21. Sataloff RT, Spiegel JR, Hawkshaw MJ. Strobovideolaryngoscopy: results and clinical value. *Annals of Otology, Rhinology and Laryngology.* 1991;100:725–727.

22. CSL Options. Retrieved June 8, 2007 from http://www.kayelemetrics. com/Product.

23. Gartner-Schmidt J. Personal communication, July 31, 2007.

24. Radionoff SL. Sound: a balancing act. *Texas Sings!* 2005;Winter:8–9.

25. Stasney CR. *Advice for Care of the Professional Voice.* Texas Voice Center Brochure; 2007.

26. Moore RJ III. *Body of Knowledge.* Houston, Tex: Body of Knowledge Inc.; 2006.

27. Roizen MF, Oz MC. *You: The Owners Manual.* New York, NY: Harper Collins Publishers; 2005.

28. Sataloff RT. *Professional Voice: The Science and Art of Clinical Care.* 2nd ed. San Diego, Calif: Singular Publishing Group; 1997:111–130.

29. Beiden D. Personal communication, July 18, 2007.

30. Radionoff SL. Is your voice tied up in knots? *Texas Sings!* 1996;Fall:14–15.

31. Rosen CA, Hathaway B, Gartner-Schmidt J, Simpson CB, Postma G, Courey M, Sataloff RT. *Clinical validation of a nomenclature paradigm for benign vocal fold lesions.* Paper presented at: 35th Annual Symposium Care of the Professional Voice, The Voice Foundation; June 4, 2006; Philadelphia, Pa.

32. Stasney CR. *Atlas of Dynamic Laryngeal Pathology.* San Diego, Calif: Singular Publishing Group; 1996.

33. Sataloff RT. Proposal for establishing a degree of doctor of philosophy in arts medicine. *Journal of Voice.* 1992;6:17–21.

Suggested Reading List

Vocal Pedagogy

A Complete Treatise on the Art of Singing: Parts 1 and 2. Ed Donald Paschke. Da Capo Press. 1984.

Singing: The Mechanism and the Technic. William Vennard. Carl Fischer. 1967.

García: The Centenarian and His Times. Sterling MacKinlay. Da Capo Press. 1976.

English, French, German and Italian Techniques of Singing. Richard Miller. Scarecrow Press. 1977.

Overtones of Bel Canto. Berton Coffin. Scarecrow Press. 1980.

The Science of Vocal Pedagogy. Ralph Appelman. Midland Press. 1986.

The Functional Unity of the Singing Voice. Barbara Doscher. Scarecrow Press. 1988.

Historical Vocal Pedagogy Classics. Berton Coffin. Scarecrow Press. 1989.

Training Tenor Voices. Richard Miller. Schirmer Books. 1993.

Choral Pedagogy. Brenda Smith and Robert T. Sataloff. Singular Publishing. 2000.

Vocalise Books

20 Vocalises. S.C. De Marchesi.G. Schirmer Publishing. 1899.

Master Vocal Exercises. Horatio Connell. Theodore Presser Company. 1927.

An Hour of Study: Exercises for the Voice (Books 1 & 2). Pauline Viardot (1821–1910. Belwin Mills Publishing. 1985.

Bel Canto: A Theoretical and Practical Vocal Method. Mathilde Marchesi. Dover. 1970.

Nicola Vaccai: Practical Method of Italian Singing. Ed Paton. G. Schirmer Inc.1975.

Voice Science/Instrumentation

Clinical Examination of Voice. Minoru Hirano. Springer-Verlag. 1981.

The Science of the Singing Voice. Johan Sundberg. Northern Illinois University Press. 1987.

Voice-Tradition and Technology: A State-of-the-Art Studio. Garyth Nair. Singular Publishing. 1999.

Clinical Measurement of Speech and Voice. Ronald J. Baken. Allyn & Bacon Press. 2000.

Clinical Speech and Voice Management: Laboratory Exercises. Robert F. Orlikoff and Ronald J. Baken. Singular Publishing. 1993.

Readings in Clinical Spectrography of Speech. Ronald J. Baken and Raymond Daniloff. Singular Publishing. 1991.

Body/Health

Blood Types BodyTypes and You. Joseph Christiano. Siloam Press. 2004.

You: The Owners Manual. Michael Roizen and Mehmet Oz. Harper Collins Publishers. 2005.

Body of Knowledge. Robert Moore III. Body of Knowledge Inc. 2006.

Vocal Health/Medical Issues

Is Your Voice Telling on You? Daniel Boone. Singular Publishing. 1991.

Voice Surgery. Wilbur J. Gould, Robert Sataloff, and Joseph Spiegel. Mosby Publishing. 1993.

Diagnosis and Treatment of Voice Disorders. John Rubin, Robert T. Sataloff, Gwen Korovin, and WJ Gould. Igaku-Shoin. 1995.

Atlas of Dynamic Laryngeal Pathology. C. Richard Stasney. Singular Publishing. 1996.

Keep your Voice Healthy. FS Brodnitz. College Hill Press. 1988.

Vocal Health and Pedagogy. Ed Robert T. Sataloff. Singular Publishing. 1998.

Voice Therapy Clinical Studies (2nd ed.). Ed. Joseph Stemple. Singular Publishing. 2000.

Vocal Health CD-ROM. J. David Garrett, Sharon L. Radionoff, Margarita Rodriguez, and C. Richard Stasney. Blue Tree Publishing. 2003.

Reflux Laryngitis and Related Disorders. Robert T. Sataloff, Donald Castell, Philip Katz, Dahlia M. Sataloff. Singular Publishing. 2003.

Arts Medicine

Professional Voice: The Science and Art of Clinical Care. 2nd ed. Robert T. Sataloff. Singular Publishing. 1997 (1st ed. 1991).

Performing Arts Medicine. Robert T. Sataloff, Alice Brandfonbrener, and Richard Ledermann. Singular Publishing. 1998 (1st ed. 1991).

Vocal Arts Medicine. Michael Benninger, Barbara Jacobson, and Alex Johnson. Thieme Publishing, 1994 .

The Performer's Voice. Michael Benninger and Thomas Murray. Plural Publishing. 2006.

Educational CD-ROMs

Blue Tree Publishing (http://www.Bluetreepublishing.com)

- Vocal Health
- Vocal Parts
- Respiration
- The Ear
- Miscellaneous others as well

Chapter 4

Private Studio Teachers/Students

$\mathscr{P}$rivate studio teaching takes place in a variety of settings and can be found in educational, religious, and private sectors. In middle school and high school settings the choir director may also teach voice or the director may engage the services of an outside voice teacher to come to the school and teach his/her students during the day. The objective for most of these students is to learn music for their choir, UIL choir festival, as well as solo and ensemble music, special school programs, and musicals. These students may also be involved in school and/or community theatre as well as religious and community choral groups.

In a college or university setting you may be contracted as an adjunct or part-time faculty or you may have a position as a full-time professor (i.e., appropriate title related to experience level). You may teach classical voice, commercial voice, or musical theatre students. If you are a full professor then you will most likely teach a course as well as have advising duties and meetings to attend. The repertoire that you teach will be based on the curriculum and program of study that your particular students are enrolled in.

In the academy setting affiliated with churches, the voice teacher is usually contracted for each teaching assignment based on need. An example of the academy setting is the Bridges Fine Arts Academy, which is affiliated with St. Luke's United Methodist Church in Houston, Texas. The objective of the voice teacher in this setting is to teach a classically based, solid vocal technique. The repertoire is classically focused but may branch into sacred music as well as musical theatre.[1] In this setting, the mission statement of the academy is to "teach the arts in many ways, and always with a 'bridge' to worship."[2] Other churches establish this setting in order to train up the next generation of music leadership in the church.[3]

In the synagogue setting the cantor often plays a dual role as a voice teacher/coach. He or she is expected to prepare candidates for Bar Mitzvahs and Bat Mitzvahs. The cantor often has quite a challenge as the charge under his or her tutelage may or may not be musically inclined. The difficulties could include vocal production and pitch issues as well as a lack of knowledge of practice skills. There may also be the added issue of problems with decoding or phonetically sounding out the Hebrew. These issues can bring about a high level of stress for the candidate, candidate's parents and cantor.[4]

In the private sector you will have the liberty to work with all ages, genres, disciplines, and levels of singers. These disciplines include, among others, (1) music educator, (2) choral participant, (3) the worship leader/cantor, (4) the professional singer (classical and commercial genres, refer to Chapter 7), and (5) the professional actor/singer (theatre/musical theatre). The objectives and repertoire for these students will be as varied as the type and number of students that you teach.

Private studio teaching of voice students includes teaching voice lessons to students that only study voice and teaching voice lessons to students that have studied and play other instruments. Prior to discussing these scenarios it is necessary to outline studio setups including studio policies as well as factors that need to be considered such as the number of students you teach.

Studio Setup

Studio policies may be predetermined or they may be flexible and are meant to establish the guidelines of the operating procedures of the studio to provide for clearly outlined expectations. Guidelines may be determined by the school, college/university, or the arts academy. The studio guideline in the private sector will be unique to each studio. Items usually covered in a studio policy include (1) attendance, (2) expectations, (3) cancellation policy, and (4) fees. Table 4–1 is an example of a University Private Studio Policy.

Studio policies in the private sector deal mainly with attendance and payment. Table 4–2 is an example of a private sector studio policy.

Along with studio policies, factors that need to be considered in regard to private studio teaching include: (1) room setup, (2) number of students in a row or per day, (3) time of lessons, (4) self-accompaniment,

> **Table 4–1.** University Private Studio Policy*

A few ground rules for voice lessons:

1. There are only four valid reasons for missing a lesson:
   a. Illness
   b. Musical Performance
   c. Bona Fide Emergency
   d. My Absence

In the case of illness, I would like as much advance notice as possible of cancellation. In the case of performance, I require three days notice. Emergencies, of course, happen when they happen. Notice may be impossible. However, if you can't notify me of an emergency before your lesson, let me know ASAP. Don't wait until the following lesson.

You are entitled to one "miss" per term for a nonvalid reason. After that your grade is affected. I do not make up lessons missed for reasons other than the above.

Point of information: My lessons schedule is occasionally disrupted by presentations/lectures or workshops. If I have to cancel your lesson I will try to give you as much notice as possible. Of course, all lessons that I miss will be made up.

2. Please bring a notebook to your lessons. Write down all exercises, useful concepts and repertoire assignments. You may record your lessons if you like.
3. You will be responsible to make a repertoire notebook of music for your accompanist and one for me.
4. To aid in learning new music you are required to:
   a. Make flashcards (index cards) of the text of your songs.
   b. Type out the text of each song on a separate sheet of paper.
      i. If foreign language a literal and poetic translation as well
   c. Make exercises of melodic patterns that recur in the music
5. If you are learning a piece in a foreign language, please know the literal translation of the text before you bring the piece to a lesson. I will not listen to a piece in a lesson unless you have translated it. Don't sing words you don't understand The following are options of collections of song and aria translations:
   a. Bernac, *The Interpretation of French Song*
   b. Coffin (Ed), *Word by Word Translations of Songs and Arias*, 2 Vols.

continues

119

Table 4–1. *continued*

c. Miller, *The Ring of Words*
d. Paquin, *Ten Cycles of Lieder*
e. Phillips, *Lieder Line by Line*

Caution: English "versions" that appear in a body of a song or aria, usually below the original text, are almost never literal translations.

6. Please note that the repertoire requirements listed in the Voice Department requirements sheet are the minimum requirement. Please don't expect the maximum grade for minimum work.
7. Except in emergencies, please do not interrupt other students' lessons to see me. My schedule is posted on my door. You are welcome to come and talk during breaks or between lessons.
8. Please don't bring food or beverages other than water to your lessons.
9. When it is time for your lesson, please knock, then come in. Don't wait for me to emerge.
10. If you need to change your regular lesson time once the term is underway, it is your responsibility, not mine, to find another student with whom to trade. Consult me only after all else fails.
11. Be sure that you know all the requirements that are expected of you for your degree plan. If you have questions do no hesitate to ask.

*Studio policy used by Dr. Sharon Radionoff at the University of Houston

---

Table 4–2. Private Sector Studio Policy

Sound Singing Institute
Office Policies

1. Payment is due when service is rendered or prepayment may be arranged in advance. Payment is accepted in the form of cash or check made out to "Sound Singing Institute." Credit Cards are *NOT* accepted at this time.

2. There is a **24-hour** cancellation policy without penalty of payment. Otherwise, you will be billed for the scheduled session.

3. Please be mindful of your speaking volume while in the waiting area as there are lessons in progress.

---

(5) vocal demonstration, and (6) use of the speaking voice. In regard to the room setup, it is important to have the space you need to accomplish your desired teaching goals as well as the items necessary to bring about an efficient and excellent experience for the student. If you choose to have the student incorporate stretching and airflow exercises on the floor then it will be necessary to have a mat and pillows accessible. If you wish to have the student demonstrate the physicality he or she uses in performance such as character movement and basic choreography, then it will be necessary to have easy mobility of mats, pillows, and student/visitor chairs. Therefore, padded folding chairs for the students and observers are recommended. For the teacher, it is important for body posture and avoiding potential physical fatigue that a padded, adjustable office chair with no arms and wheels is used in lieu of a piano bench. This way the teacher will have freedom of movement to observe the student from many angles and positions. Another factor which allows for full observation of the student is the use and placement of mirrors. It is also beneficial to have easy access to visual teaching aids, models, support cards, charts, and so forth. One last important issue is having some type of recording and playback system setup in the studio should the student wish to record the session. Most students today request a CD recording format and not cassette tape format. Some students also request videotape availability (Figure 4-1).

It will be important to know what effect the number of students in a row has on the physical demands of the teacher. This will need to be adjusted depending on each teacher. All teachers, however, need to make time for personal physical stretching and movement during the day. In regard to setting up the time of lessons in the private sector, the teacher will need to be sensitive to the school and work schedules of their students. It may be beneficial to schedule work days from Tuesday through Saturday and take Mondays off. The lesson times for other scenarios will be somewhat flexible but will most likely, overall, be determined by the school, academy, or synagogue schedules.

It is important to make it very clear to any potential and first-time students whether or not you choose to self-accompany their lessons. There are pros and cons of each stance. If you choose to accompany, how accomplished your keyboard skills are will have an effect on how well you are able to focus on the technical and musical aspects of the student. Also, the placement of the keyboard and the effect on the efficiency of your body alignment may affect your physical health

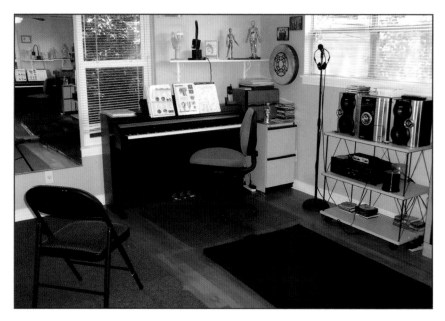

Figure 4–1. Studio room set-up of the Sound Singing Institute, Houston, Texas.

and your vocal health. On the positive side, you will be able to nego-tiate the singer through many issues and exercises if you have adequate keyboard skills along with good theory skills. Some of these services may include transposition of keys for helping students choose appro-priate keys (although there are transposing keyboards). Furthermore, if a teacher has accompaniment skills, a student may be able to attend more lessons if they do not also need to hire an accompanist. Another option that is available is the use of prerecorded tracks to practice and perform with.

Teachers frequently use vocal demonstration during a voice les-son. Although this may seem like the quickest way to get the point across, it has the potential to cause problems. If the student is young or of the same voice category as the teacher, he or she is in danger of trying to mimic the sound quality of the teacher in order to please the teacher. This may not be in the best interest of the student as he or she may be creating compensatory behavior to create the desired sound instead of using his or her healthy natural anatomic configura-tion. Also, if the teacher's head or neck is in an inefficient position when demonstrating, then there is the possibility of vocal fatigue and potentially serious vocal problems in the future. It is certainly appropriate to demonstrate to teach a warm-up but another thing to "sing along" with a student while he or she does the exercise. Furthermore, although some teachers regard themselves to be the authority in regard to stylistic interpretation of a song, another technique that students can use for musicality and interpretation ideas is to listen to several different recordings of the same song by different performers.

The last factor discussed is use of the speaking voice. While this is the last item, it is certainly not the least important. In fact, as outlined in Chapter 5, it is noted that music educators use their voices all day long, whether for instruction, discipline, or demonstration. Voice teachers are no different. There is a high demand for voice use as many voice teachers perform as well as teach.

Singers think about and train their singing technique in order to be excellent performers. In fact, efficient technique is critical to healthy vocal survival. The same holds true for speaking. Technique for speaking includes such issues as pitch, resonance, breath control (managed airflow), rate of speed, and volume level. Remember that the same instrument is used for both speaking and singing. A very common problem with teachers is that they often speak with too low of a pitch. This can be the result of trying to sound more authoritative or from speaking when frustrated or it can be from diminished airflow due to using "therapy voice" (speaking softly and dropping the pitch using laryngeal resonance). Speaking with too low a pitch can lead to hyperfunction or muscle tension dysphonia (MTD) as outlined in Chapter 3. It would be highly beneficial for all teachers to receive training in their speaking voices. Issues that must be considered include: (1) physical body alignment, (2) technique of speaking, and (3) use of the speaking voice. As discussed above in regard to demonstrating, if the body is in an inefficient position while talking then there is potential for vocal fatigue and harm. When we sing we know that we must have excellent technique for longevity of voice use. It is the same for speaking! There must be a balance of the necessary systems (power source/pitch source/sound quality shaper), as discussed in Chapter 1, in order to have freedom and flexibility of voicing.

Sometimes singers also teach other things such as university classes, religious classes, or other instrumental lessons and the same issues of speaking when teaching hold true here. Also be sure not to talk over other voices or instruments (Figure 4-2). Additional factors

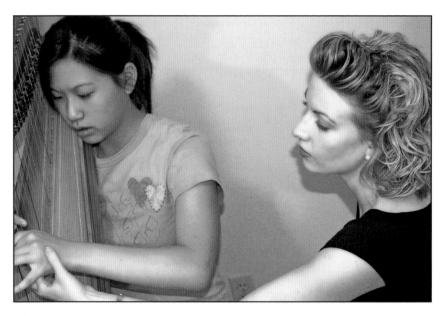

Figure 4–2. Singer/Harpist Stacey Weber teaching Amy Chan.

to be considered other than use of the voice during actual teaching include (1) amount of telephone time and technique while on the phone, (2) yelling, and (3) speaking voice use at home.

Giving a Voice Lesson

Introduction

As noted in Chapter 3, Richard Miller states that the voice teacher should do no harm and that the analysis and plan for training should be based on current research and information of the instrument, not subjective imagery.[5,6] An example of subjective imagery would be "imagine that you feel the airflow shooting out the top of your head like whirling blades of a helicopter."

The voice teacher's goals postanalysis are to: (1) set up a plan of study, (2) teach and apply concepts with the technical tools needed to carry out the plan, and (3) mentor and encourage. Common questions/

issues that are brought up by a student when he or she first meets a voice teacher include: (1) How can I increase my range? (2) How can I increase my vocal power? (3) How can I sing longer phrases? Oh and by the way . . . (4) how many lessons will it take?

It seems that there are four badges of honor that all singers love to wear. They include (1) how high (or low), (2) how long, (3) how loud, and (4) how fast.

Although the above goals are worthy to attain, remember that the teacher sets the pace or "tone" of the environment. It is important to be sensitive to the mood of the student and to allow the session to be guided by what the singer brings to the lesson in terms of preparation and how the voice/body responds on a given day.

Getting Acquainted and Diagnostics

When you see a student for the first time it is important for both the teacher and the student to have a get-acquainted time. This includes talking to the student about past experiences with music and singing such as (1) ensemble participation—voice type and part sung, (2) previous voice teachers—exercises and songs, and (3) playing of other instruments. Other pertinent questions include: (1) What do they want to do with music, (2) Why do they want to study singing, (3) What do they like about their voice, (4) What do they think that they need to work on, (5) What kind of music do they like to listen to and sing, and (6) Do they sing in other languages.[7]

After the get-acquainted time it is time to analyze the singer's voice. This can be done with two steps. First, as outlined in Chapter 3, use the 5-note ascending/descending scale to go up and down by half steps to listen for (1) the total range of the singer (Physiologic Frequency Range of Phonation/Musical Frequency Range of Phonation), (2) tessitura, (3) voice quality, and (4) technical deficits (Figure 4-3).

The technical issues to be covered include body issues of (1) stance/posture, (2) head/neck position, (3) tongue position, (4) jaw position, and (5) oral cavity opening. Breathing issues to examine include checking if they use (1) abdominal/diaphragmatic, (2) thoracic, (3) clavicular, (4) shallow, and/or (5) rapid breathing. Further questions in regard to breathing include (1) is the breath audible—which often means tension, (2) is there excessive abdominal movement or tension, and (3) is the breath flowing freely? Breath support issues to

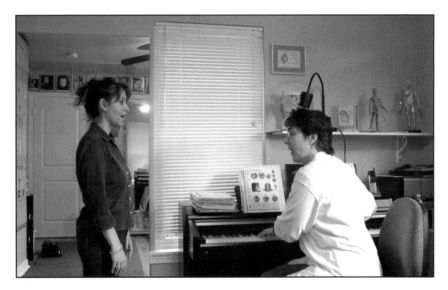

Figure 4-3. Debbie Fancher, Contemporary Christian Artist/Worship leader.

examine include (1) effective versus ineffective method, (2) deficient, (3) late, or (4) use of the inverse pressure method. Range and registration issues include (1) smooth transition versus voice breaks, (2) mechanisms equally developed, (3) lack of coordination or development, (4) usable range (short or sufficient), (5) is range/repertoire that they are singing suitable for the voice. Tension points to be aware of include (1) forehead, (2) tongue, (3) jaw—clenching/jutting/restricting, (4) neck, (5) strap muscles, (6) vertical laryngeal position, (7) shoulders, (8) ribs, and (9) abdominal musculature. One last issue to monitor is vibrato. If it is present, is it appropriate, and if it is not present is it appropriate?

The second step of analysis includes having the singer sing a song in whatever style he or she is comfortable with. It is important that students be told prior to the lesson to come prepared to do this. If the student has never had a lesson before then the singer can sing a hymn, folk song, or Happy Birthday. After the analysis is done, it is important to discuss the findings with the student in a positive, constructive way. Discuss exercises that they have used from previous teachers or choir directors and integrate what you feel is appropriate. Next, it is time to give feedback and outline the plan of study. It is important to choose and decide which three main points to focus on—there will be many things that you see but you do not want to overload the student. It is typical for the beginning teacher to try to impart all of the information at once. The only thing that this will accomplish is to frustrate the student.

If there is time in the first session, it is also important to discuss vocal health issues. These can include general body health and drying agents. The basics as outlined in Chapter 3 for general body health include the issues of (1) hydration, (2) diet, (3) rest, and (4) exercise. The basics as outlined in Chapter 3 for drying agents include the issues of (1) caffeine, (2) alcohol, and (3) diuretics.

When you begin teaching it is beneficial to journal thoughts and responses after each lesson. The following is an idea of where to begin: Start with an introductory statement about each student after the first lesson. Begin the statement with a brief account of what happened in the lesson. Then go on to discuss your impressions. As best you can tell after one hearing, what type of voice is this? What did you see and hear? What are your preliminary impressions of the student's strengths and weaknesses—technical, musical, and expressive? What do you think this student needs to help him or her grow and improve? What kinds of exercises or technical ideas do you think you will try with this student?[7]

After the introductory statement, write impressions about each succeeding lesson. Start with a brief description of the lesson, then move on to any ideas or impressions that you think are relevant. How did the student respond to your instruction? Which ideas or expressions seemed to have the most positive impact? Do you find the student easy or difficult to teach? Why? Do you have doubts about anything you are doing? What are they? What aspects of teaching do you feel you need to know more about to resolve those doubts? Did any new thoughts occur to you as you heard the student this time? Did anything surprise you? How did you feel about the lesson? Also after each lesson describe what you did, if you will change anything, and what the future plans are.[7]

You do not need to answer all of these questions. These are simply points of departure for discussing your work. Besides providing a record of the lessons, the object of these journal entries is to help spark your imagination as a teacher and to sharpen your perception of what is occurring in your lessons. So, it is important that you write about your own concerns and questions.[7]

Other questions that you can ask yourself include: Which concepts, expressions, or approaches seemed to work best with students? Do your perceptions of your students change as time progresses? Which insights, understandings, or experiences contribute to your improvement as a teacher? In which ways have you not succeeded? Have you learned anything from your failures? What do you think your strengths and weaknesses are as a teacher? Do you enjoy teaching? What do you like most about it? What do you like least? Does your experience as a teacher help you understand your own voice better? Does it help you understand yourself better? Again, this is not an all-inclusive list of questions to be answered completely, but points of departure for thought and growth.[7]

The Second Lesson

Now the fun begins! It is important to remember that the singer is an athlete. Therefore, it is important to understand and have an awareness of the body (which is the voice) and how it naturally functions. You have to be aware of how the body works for breathing naturally before you can move to the highest athletic level. It is important to begin on exhalation as outlined in the airflow exercises in Chapter 2. Remember that if you begin by exhaling whatever breath you have in your body, you will get to a point where you must release to allow breath to come in. This will help the student to avoid the issue of "tanking up" and overworking for inhalation. Remember that inhalation is always an active process that must occur for us to stay alive—we don't have to work to make breath come in—we must allow it to come in. Below, a 3-part vocalizing plan is outlined.

Vocalizing Plan (Consult Chapter 2 for exercise details)

Phase One/Voice Preparation/Balancing
- Stress Release Exercises
- Relaxation/Airflow Exercises
- Descending APS Exercises
- Tone Balancing Exercise

Phase Two
- Systems Alignment
- Building block
- Multitasking

- Song patterns
- Chanting
  - Use of medium dynamics
  - Use of narrow range
  - Use of few vowel changes

Phase Three
- Introduce/Increase difficulty of exercises
  - Length of exercise
  - Range of exercise
  - Vowel changes
  - Extreme dynamics

It is easy to get caught in a trap of being in a hurry when teaching. Be sure that you do not confuse handing out information with teaching. Teaching is guiding through concepts with exercises, not merely giving out lists of exercises to practice. You will need to develop the sense of when to "push" the student and when to back off. Also don't be in a hurry to classify a voice type because many voices don't reveal themselves until a later time. Remember to keep notes on each lesson. You may feel like you are teaching the same concept for many weeks in a row—remember we didn't get to where we are overnight nor will we change overnight![7]

Lessons Continued

Vocalizing

If during the vocalizing process there is tightness of sound this relates to body tension which will also cause airflow tension or lack of freedom of airflow. Exercises that may be beneficial here are included from Chapter 2:

- Descending slides, wavy slides, and roller coaster slides
- Descendings
- Pitch games

You may also notice other extraneous tension which is energy that does not belong. Places of tension may include (1) neck and shoulders, (2) jaw tension, (3) pharyngeal tension, (4) tongue tension and overall body tension. For the neck and shoulders there are passive and active exercises that may be beneficial. The passive exercises consist of using your own arm weight to help release the neck tension. An example of this exercise would be:

- Clasp your palms together and place them at the nape of your neck.
- Allow your head to roll forward so that your chin is close to/or touching your chest
- Allow your elbows to rest together at the center of your body
  - Be sure not to hold your breath. It is important to do each exercise two times. The first time gets rid of tension and the second time you get the stretch. Carry out each repetition for 40 to 60 seconds.

Active exercises on the other hand consist of physically moving your muscles. Exercises for this grouping include:

- roll head and neck in a slow frontal semicircle
- free floating head (pen on top of head making designs on the ceiling)
- shoulder rolls
- raise shoulders up and then let down
- rag doll

Jaw tension release exercises may include:

- Massage jaw
- blub blub
- Head back, mouth hang open, bring head forward and keep mouth hanging
- jah, jah, joh, joh
- Chewing

Pharyngeal tension—often includes tongue tension and is often related to overworking to "create" a certain space for a vowel sound or for a quality of sound:

- Yawn sigh
- Use diphthongs
- Work voice through naturalness of speech
- M word list, short word list, sentences with nasalants

Tongue tension—often includes jaw tension/clenching/articulation

- ■ Roll the 'r'
- ■ Blah Blah
- ■ Phrase to promote independence of tongue and jaw
- ■ Patter songs
- ■ "Lips teeth tip of the tongue"
  - ○ single note, 54321 pattern

Body tension—rigidity of posture

- ■ add arm movement
- ■ add body sway[7]

General Concepts

When balancing and working patterns for sound, there are a series of concepts to pay attention to. There are (a) tone choices, (b) consonant choices, and (c) vowel choices. Within tone choices it is most efficient to begin with (a) a single note in a comfortable pitch area, and then (b) move to stepwise patterns, (c) next skipping patterns, and (d) lastly agility patterns. These patterns are discussed in detail in Chapter 2.

Within consonant choices it will be important to assess whether the concept needed is to (1) move airflow, (2) feel a safety control, (3) create the environment of a natural ease of frontal resonance, and/or (4) end sound with air and not with glottal squeezing.[8]

- ■ Move Airflow
  - ○ Level 1:
    - • Begin with Unvoiced consonant first
      - ▪ f, s, sh
  - ○ Level 2:
    - • Add l or w (e.g. Fl, Fw, woom, loom. Woop, loop)
      - ▪ Use l: The tongue base will release some tension when the tongue tip touches up on the hard palate (alveolar ridge)
      - ▪ Use of w: the lips come apart for a "w" which aids in the sound releasing out of the mouth

- Use Voiced Consonants
  - v, z, zh
- Safety Control (psychological feeling)
  - Use of the plosive b
    - Use of the plosive b: In order to produce a "b" air pressure builds up behind a pair of closed lips and it is unnecessary to push or shove airflow to create this production.
- Natural ease of frontal resonance (otherwise known as head voice resonance or resonant voice by SLPs)
  - Use of the nasalant consonant m
    - Use of the nasalant m: It is not necessary to push sound forward in order to produce an "m" all one has to do is close the lips.
- End sound with air and no squeeze at the glottis ending with
  - Use of p and t
    - First choice: use p because the tongue position can stay behind the bottom teeth for the production of the "p."
    - Second choice: use t. This choice can be more difficult because the tongue moves and there is the possibility of pressing the tongue into palate.[8]

Within vowel choice the concept is to create the environment of a space that will enhance verticality of molar position/jaw release without fighting air and space for sound. The vowel choices /u/ and /o/, aid in resonance tract efficiency. /u/ is a round/small vowel tube and /o/ is an oblong vertical tube.

- Vowel Choices
  - Begin with /u/ and /o/
    - Use of /u/ and /o/: These choices aid in creating vertical resonance tract space. The use of /u/ is a small vowel space and helps to produce sound without fighting air and sound for space
  - Move to other vowels
    - We often tend to overwork for space for vowel sounds. See how little you have to work to produce an accurate vowel. Remember that vowels are produced by the shape of the tongue primarily (and rounded lips for /u/ and /o/).[8]

Singers Who Play Other Instruments

Many singers also play a variety of instruments. Along with singing in choirs they are often members of a marching band, concert band, jazz band, symphony orchestra, religious orchestra/band, praise band, or community band. When a student is a music education major in college if voice is the primary instrument then piano is most often the automatic secondary major. It is a "bonus" for the university if the student is an accomplished instrumentalist as well. Music education majors will also be required to take group/class lessons of a variety of instruments. For singers who play other instruments, there are unique issues with embouchure (basically mouth/lip/jaw position) and body alignment which can affect easy, balanced phonation. These issues are different for brass and woodwind instruments and there are also differences within each group, respectively. There are also issues in regard to guitar/keyboard training/playing and singing. It seems that there is a correlation between what instrument one has trained first and the brain's association with a checklist of "I do such and such for music." Thus, an aspect of training for a brass or woodwind instrument such as musculature for the "embouchure" can trickle into what we do when we sing. Some call this muscle memory, some call it learned behavior—the label really doesn't matter—the activity is what it is.

Brass

For brass instruments there are specific potential pitfalls which include: (1) jaw position moving forward for a proper embouchure, (2) mouth/lip position for the embouchure, (3) glottal tension, and (4) laryngeal tension.

In Figure 4-4 we see an example of efficient body position and embouchure for playing trombone. In Figure 4-5 we see a close-up view of the jaw position and the mouth/lip position needed for excellence in trombone playing. Notice the pulled back lips and tight chin position. Although there may be jaw and lip position issues that have the potential to affect what a musician does when singing, the glottis and larynx configuration while playing trombone (Figure 4-6) is more singing transferable than the glottal/laryngeal configuration while playing the trumpet

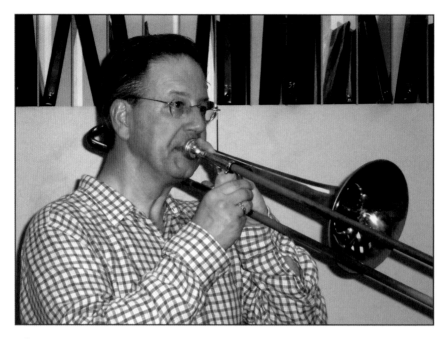

Figure 4–4. Lee Poquette, Director of Music/Trombonist, West University Baptist Church, Houston, Texas.

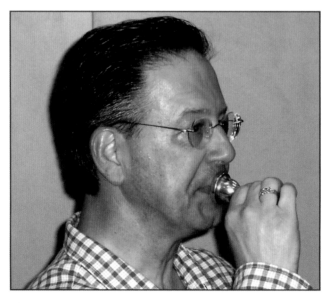

Figure 4–5. Lee Poquette, Close-up view of the trombone embouchure.

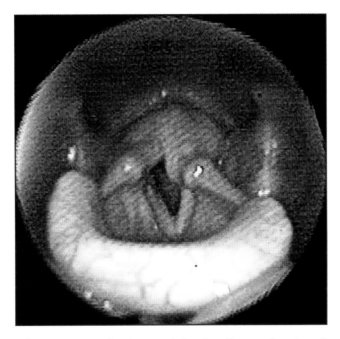

Figure 4-6. The larynx/glottis of a professional trombonist.

When playing the trumpet, as seen in the stroboscopy picture of Figure 4-7, the front two-thirds of the vocal folds are together and there is a keyhole opening in the back of the glottis. Also notice that the false vocal folds on both sides are coming in toward midline. This configuration provides an aesthetically pleasing sound for this professional symphonic trumpeter, however, if carried into singing this configuration would be called MTD (muscle tension dysphonia). It is actually similar to what we see in voicing a stage whisper (Figure 4-8). Review and compare normal for trumpet playing (see Figure 4-7) with normal for singing (Figure 4-9). In Figure 4-10, we see that the false vocal folds almost completely cover over the glottis in a trumpeter with unhealthy or bad technique.

It is interesting to note that many private and public schools offer private instrumental lessons to students starting in the fourth and fifth grades and one of the instruments that is most often taught is the trumpet. Some students start playing the trumpet as young as nine years of age. There are research studies which demonstrate the

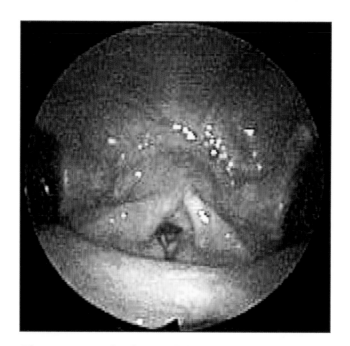

Figure 4-7. The larynx/glottis of a professional symphony trumpeter.

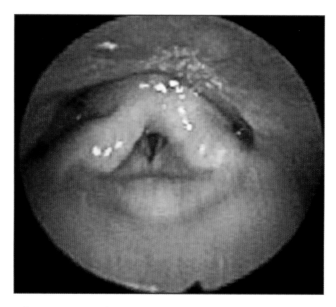

Figure 4-8. The larynx/glottis configuration of a stage whisper.

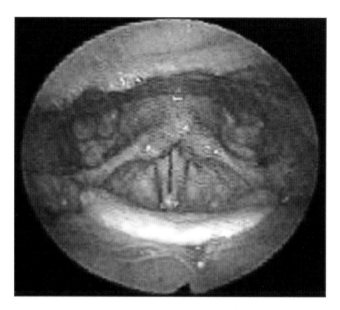

Figure 4–9. The larynx/pharynx normal configuration while singing.

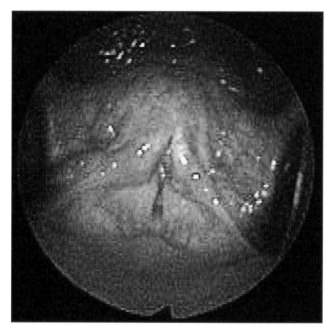

Figure 4–10. The larynx/glottis configuration of bad trumpet technique.

potential problems of young students playing an instrument such as the trumpet prior to tissues developing fully. In a study by Stasney, Beaver, and Rodriguez,[9] the issue of a potential "laryngocele" or blowout of the larynx in a young brass player is discussed. High notes demand high internal throat pressure which may result in a blowout. This is essentially a herniation in the laryngeal tissue and its appearance may resemble a neck mass if it is external. There are also internal laryngoceles which are limited to the interior of the larynx.[10]

In Figure 4-11 we see an internal view of the pharynx via stroboscopy of a French hornist. Notice how elevated the epiglottis and tongue are. They are so high that it is impossible to see the vocal folds. Again, although this configuration provides for an esthetically pleasing sound for a professional symphony hornist, it would be considered unhealthy for a singer. It is important to mention that the article by Stasney et al. stated that the French horn requires the greatest throat pressure of all pitches and instruments that were tested.[9]

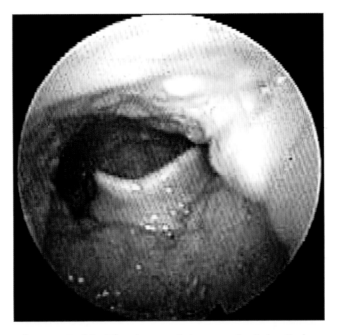

Figure 4-11. The larynx/pharynx/epiglottis/ tongue configuration of a professional French hornist.

Woodwind

Just as brass instruments have a set of potential pitfalls for the singer so do the woodwind instruments. Some of the woodwinds specific pitfalls include: (1) neck/glottal tension, (2) jaw position moving back for the embouchure, (3) chin tucking for the clarinet and oboe, (4) high tongue position for the oboe, (5) upper lip pursing and over the lower lip for the flute, (6) the bottom lip rolling over the bottom teeth and biting into the mouthpiece with the top teeth for the clarinet, and (7) the head/neck position often at an angle for playing the flute.

In Figure 4-12, because the chin must be tucked for playing the oboe, we see the arytenoid cartilages, part of the epiglottis and tongue and we also see a very small bit of the opening between the vocal folds at the posterior (back) of the glottis prior to the oboist playing. In Figure 4-13, once the oboist is playing, due to the chin tuck and the tongue riding high, it is impossible to see the vocal folds.

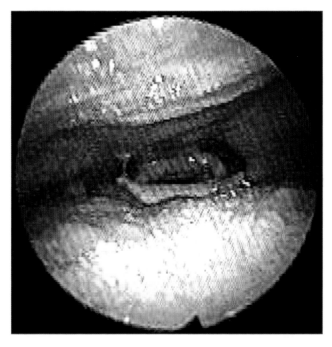

Figure 4-12. The larynx/pharynx configuration of a professional oboist prior to playing.

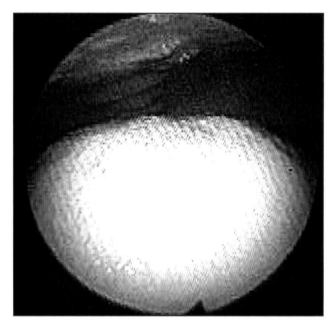

Figure 4-13. The pharynx/tongue configuration of a professional oboist while playing.

Guitar/Keyboard

There are several factors that are key to helping a singer who also plays guitar and/or keyboard while singing. It is crucial to healthy vocal production and longevity to pay specific attention to the head/neck position (Figure 4-14). The singer who plays guitar or keyboard while singing often feels the need to protrude the head forward and to elevate the head toward the microphone. It seems that although using a boom stand microphone does help, there is still an inclination to use the inefficient head/neck position. Another issue to analyze with the dual activity of singing and playing the guitar is how one holds the guitar (Figure 4-15). The body position of shoulders, rib cage, and upper torso, if inefficient, has the potential to adversely affect breathing. There are also issues of different weights of guitars. It is important to evaluate the upper body strength of the player and the shape of the spine in regard to strap recommendations. There are actually choices in guitar straps. Most performers who play and sing use a shoulder strap; however there is a neck strap available.

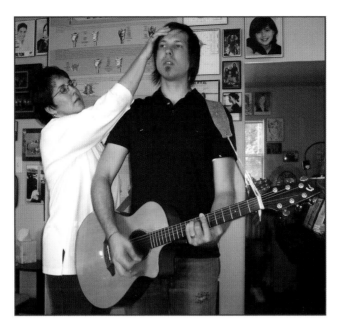

Figure 4–14. Aaron Rodriguez, Lakewood Youth Music Ministry, Lakewood Church, Houston, Texas.

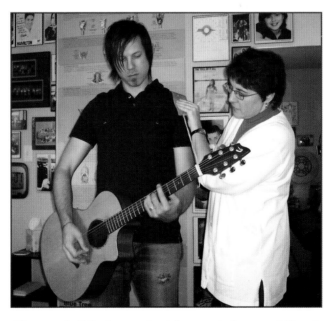

Figure 4–15. Aaron Rodriguez, Lakewood Youth Music Ministry, Lakewood Church, Houston, Texas.

Harp

It is interesting to note that while the harpist is not using any voicing, there may be skeletal issues that occur which have the potential to effect the voice. The arm position of the harpist can be very tiring to the shoulders, back, and neck. In this instance the harpist uses therapy exercises to help her body stay as supple as possible. She recognizes the connection between skeleton, specifically shoulders/back and neck to freedom and agility of the voice. Also the sedentary position while playing has the potential to keep the body/breathing in a still position (Figure 4–16). Therefore, this student also recognizes the importance of relaxation and airflow exercises along with slides and descendings as outlined in Chapter 2.

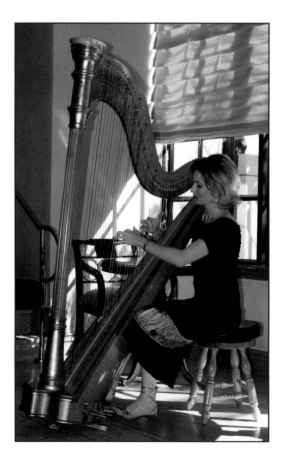

Figure 4-16. Stacey Weber, Harpist, performing for tea at a downtown hotel in Houston.

Conclusion

The issues mentioned in this chapter are relevant regardless of the style of music or the performance setting. The desired end result is to create an aesthetic, musical experience of communication. Ideally, this will be achieved with an efficient vocal system to enable longevity and freedom from fatigue and potential vocal disorders.

Acknowledgments. The author thanks Stacey Weber, Debbie Fancher, Lee Poquette, and Aaron Rodriguez for permission for Figures in order: 4-2, and 4-16, 4-3, 4-4, and 4-5, and 4-14, and 4-15.
    The author thanks Dr. C. Richard Stasney (Texas Voice Center) for permission to use Figures 4-6 through 4-13

References

1. Bridges Fine Arts Academy. Retrieved August 24, 2007 from http://www.stlukesmethodist.org/programs/arts/bridges.aspx.
2. Murrow R. Personal communication, August 23, 2007.
3. Li WCS. *Prevaling Principles and Practices in Church-Affiliated Music Academies of Selected Southern Baptist Churches in the United States* [D.M.A. dissertation]. University of Houston, Texas, 2001. Available from: ProQuest Digital Dissertations. Retrieved August 26, 2007, Publication Number: AAT 3035542.
4. Dorf D. Personal communication, August 23, 2007.
5. Miller R. The singing teacher in the age of voice science. In: Sataloff RT, ed. *Professional Voice: The Science and Art of Clinical Care*. New York, NY: Raven Press; 1991:375-380.
6. Radionoff SL. *Objective Measures of Vocal Production During the Course of Singing Study* [Doctoral dissertation]. Michigan State University; 1996. Available from: ProQuest Digital Dissertations. Retrieved September 8, 2007, Publication Number: AAT 9631333.
7. Radionoff SL. *Undergraduate Performance Pedagogy*. Course syllabus, University of Houston, Houston, Tex; Fall 2000.
8. Radionoff SL. Pop culture music trends: Part two. *Texas Sings!* 2007; Spring;10-11,17.
9. Stasney CR, Beaver ME, Rodriguez M. Hypopharyngeal pressure in brass musicians. *Medical Problems of Performing Artists.* 2003;18,4:153-155.
10. Isaacson G, Sataloff RT. Bilateral laryngoceles in a young trumpet player: Case report. *Ear, Nose and Throat Journal.* 2000;79:272-274.

Chapter 5

Music Educators

The field of music education requires high-end voice use that starts when the bell rings and continues to the end of the day without any real voice-off or voice-rest time. Music educators can have up to 8 classes back to back per day (including double class loads of 60 to 70 students). There may be a scheduled lunch hour, but teachers often have to "serve" lunch duty. Other voice use requirements can include bus duty after school or hall duty as well. The potential is high for breeding hyperfunction (muscular tension dysphonia).[1]

Music educators use voice for instruction, demonstration, and discipline. Therefore, they switch back and forth between speaking and singing many times during a single class period. Unfortunately, the luxury of possessing one larynx for singing and one for speaking is not available. What does this mean for the music educator? It means that speaking habits must be as pristine as possible to ensure vocal survival. This, however, is usually not the case.[1]

It is common for music educators to demonstrate the following speaking habits during conversational speech: (1) excessively low pitch, (2) low airflow, (3) harsh glottal attacks, (4) laryngeal resonance, and (5) pushed or pressed voice. These technical faults often occur as a result of the teacher trying to sound more authoritative and stern. These speaking habits then bleed into even the best singing techniques. Common singing problems include: 1) loss of range (usually upper), (2) pushed or pressed chest voice, (3) strained head voice, (4) loss of flexibility, and (5) hoarseness. Remember, we only have one larynx. Therefore, what we do when we are not singing will directly affect what we do when we sing. It is critical that the music educator who experiences difficulty undergo both speech therapy and singing voice training.[1]

Typically music educators do one or more of the following: (1) classroom teaching, (2) direct traditional ensembles and ensembles with choreography in the school setting, (3) direct a church choir, (4) have a worship leader position, (5) have a cantor position, (6) have a paid section leader position, (7) teach private lessons, and (8) personally perform.[1] Some of these different situations are discussed in detail below and others in corresponding chapters.

Additional considerations in regard to specific teaching duties include (1) class behavioral rules, (2) low/nonverbal means of discipline, (3) number of classes back to back, (4) size of classes, (5) classroom aide, and (6) assistant teacher. It will be much more efficient for and easier on the teacher if the class rules of behavior are laid out at the beginning of the school year. It is also beneficial if the students have some ownership of the class rules (of course, this is age governed). Also, write the rules on a poster board and put in plain sight for all to see. New teachers must remember that they need to be a teacher first and a friend to the students second. When discipline is necessary, it is vocally smart to use both low and nonverbal means such as a bell, hand-clap, piano chord, cutoff cue (etc.), and put stickers on a chart with the appropriate student name—consequences for actions!

It is important to discuss with the administration what the district and school rules are for number of classes that you will teach back to back as well as the size of classes. It is very difficult to teach a double class of first graders (up to 60 students) without the help of a classroom aide. It really becomes babysitting without much teaching of information being disseminated. If you are in a large district and teach middle school or high school choral music you may either be the head director and have an assistant or you may be an assistant to the head director. If you are the head director you will do a great service to your assistant and yourself if you have written preparatory checklists, have written out a list of expectations, and discuss things that may seem logical and common sense to you.

Classroom Teaching

Teaching Space: Dedicated Physical Space

There are many variables that must be considered in setting up the classroom for teaching that will allow for vocal health on the part of the music educator. What is the size of the room? Do you have "built-in" riser steps? Do you have a flat surface? Is the floor carpeted or linoleum surfaced? Is it large to accommodate a double-size classroom such that you need a microphone? Do you use AV aids such as videos, DVDs or CDs and do you talk over them? Do you have an upright or grand piano or a keyboard?

- The physical room interior will have to be taken into consideration when determining how to set up the room layout. Some things will be a given (such as built-in riser steps), and some things you can experiment with.
- In a large size room, especially if it is carpeted, you will need to use a microphone. There are many hands-free microphones available such as the "collar mic" by Anchor Audio in California so that you do not have to feel constrained.
- Instead of talking over audiovisual aids make use of call charts. You can make simple charts using a poster board and listing what you want to "call attention" to with a number next to it. This will save your voice as well as allow all students to know/hear what you want them to know.
- The positioning of the piano, whether it is an upright or a grand, can have a dramatic effect on both vocal health and effectiveness of teaching.

Teaching Space: Roving Cart

A roving cart with a keyboard on top presents a variety of potential problems. Some of the issues include (1) the height of the cart—is it fixed or adjustable? (2) the size of the keyboard—is it a full 88-key keyboard or 76 or less? What is the actual size of the keys? (3) are you standing to play? What is your arm position? This has the potential to affect forearms, wrists, fingers, and shoulders. You must be sure to guard against positioning that may lead to carpal tunnel syndrome.

- Be sure that the height of the cart with the keyboard on it is appropriate for proper arm position for playing the piano. If you are using an adjustable cart this is an easy fix, but if it is not adjustable then buy a cart that is of appropriate height.
- You can get by with a keyboard that has 76 keys but be sure that the keys are actual piano size keys. If the keys are smaller

you will compromise good technique and predispose your-self to potential physical hand/wrist problems.

■ Standing to play is not necessarily a bad thing; however, fatigue can set in after several classes in a row. It would be more body friendly to sit on a stool so that physical weariness will not overtake good posture and cause vocal problems (this is discussed in more detail in the scenarios below).

Teaching Scenarios

In the following sections I have outlined some common scenarios that music educators often encounter. These scenarios may be familiar to the music educator from either personal experience or recognition. Each scenario has corresponding sections entitled "red flags" and "problem solvers." The red flags sections refer to potential pitfalls that commonly occur in the given scenario. The problem solvers sections may either help resolve existing vocal problems, or avert potential problems. These issues must be monitored to sustain vocal health as a music educator.[2]

Level: Elementary

Scenario 1. You are an elementary school music educator. Perhaps you sit on the floor with your kindergarten and/or first grade class.

Red Flags: What is your upper torso/sternum position? Are you arching the small of your lower back? (If you are then your abdominal muscles are contracted to keep this posture and cannot be used for exhalation of airflow for singing). Is your head/neck posture in a neutral position or is it elevated and/or protruded/poking out? Is the base of your head/neck at the base of your skull compressed downward? Is your chin tucked down and in? If you have answered yes to any of these head/neck questions then you are impeding the ease of your airflow and sound production.

Problem Solvers: Music educators in this scenario typically create compensations to achieve the desired sound. The most common compensation is to use excessive muscular tension in the extrinsic laryngeal muscles (muscles on the outside of your larynx or neck muscles) to counterbalance for poor breath support or control. Practice your lesson plans while sitting on the floor and monitor your posture, breath flow/support, and resonance.[2]

Scenario 2. You are an elementary music educator who teaches a double class without an assistant. You feel like you are an entertainer instead of a teacher. If you have no microphone, then you most likely feel the need to loudly project the voice. You are also trying to keep class discipline and teach music at the same time. Because of this, you exude a high energy level of excitement to keep the students involved.

Red Flags: In an effort to create energy are you tensing your abdomen and contracting the most important muscles for singing exhalation even before using them for breath support/ control? Is your energy dispersing up and out instead of keeping body weight centered down and using your abdomen as the "control panel" (discussed in Chapter 2 sections on posture and breathing)? Other problems include: rate of speech increase, talking and singing a phrase that is too long for good vocal health, overenunciating (thus making myriad harsh glottal attacks or chewing the words with your jaw), and projecting the voice by pushing from the throat instead of using the balance of breath, phonation, and resonance. Your "systems balance" is totally out of whack!

Problem Solvers: Practice your lesson plans specifically for pacing, breath flow, resonance, and energy level. Use a microphone when teaching. There are several excellent types available such as lapel or collar microphones.[2]

Scenario 3. You are an elementary music educator and you teach with an upright piano positioned in front of your class (you accompany all of your own classes). You either sit on a regular piano bench or stand.

Red Flags: In order to see your students over the piano, have you elevated and protruded your head/neck position? Also, is your upper torso/sternum position collapsed and are you arching the small of your lower back? Are the abdominal muscles that you need for active exhalation already contracted even before breathing for singing? Do you proceed to vocally demonstrate and teach by rote while in this body posture?

Problem Solvers: Sit on a stool. This will put you in a better line of vision with your students. It will also allow you to use a healthy head/neck position and better upper torso/sternum and back position. In turn, you will be able to release and use your abdominal muscles for singing breath support. If you have a small enough class, you may wish to have your students come around the piano.[2]

Level: Middle School/Junior High School

Scenario. In this level the music educator often teaches a variation of a music appreciation class. Often students enrolled in this class need an elective and they think that this will be an easy grade. The issues of class control and student involvement can be very difficult in this situation.

Red Flags: Do you feel the need to yell to assert authority? This can either be done by raising the volume and pitch or by pushing the pitch very low.

Problem Solvers: Lay down ground rules at the beginning of the year. You can even have the students involved in setting up the classroom rules. If you are a new teacher it is very important that you do not try to be the student's friend. It is much better to start out a new year with more structure and strictness and then relax the environment later. It is very difficult, if not impossible, to try to become more strict in the middle of the school year. Other helpful hints include (1) use a series of merits and demerits, (2) use group project time, and (3) implement the Stop and Wait rule (literally telling them that you will wait till they stop misbehaving).

Level: High School

Scenario. The classroom experience at the high school level usually entails teaching a music theory and/or sight-singing class. You may also include in the curriculum composition experience. Therefore, the students enrolled in this class will most likely be there because of interest and not just for an easy credit. This will ease the burden of class control. This classroom setting does not typically pose problems out of the ordinary.

Choral Conducting

Introduction

Along with classroom teaching music educators often direct both traditional ensembles and show or jazz choirs with choreography as well. Sometimes the dedicated physical space is not exactly what you had in mind. It may actually be a stage in a gymnasium while gym classes are going on at the same time. It may be a small space with carpeting that is acoustically inadequate.

Another issue is that of self-monitoring. Have you ever argued with someone about something that they've done but weren't able to see themselves do? Imagine that multiplied by 10 to 20 students in a rehearsal for choreography where there are no mirrors. This can also happen in the traditional ensemble when talking about posture and technique.

A final consideration is the number of extra rehearsals due to contests like solo and ensemble festivals. This puts a heavy burden on the teacher's time schedule. How do you organize your time during the day so that you can accomplish what you need to accomplish?

Level: Middle School/Junior High School/ High School

Traditional

Scenario 1. You are a middle school or high school choir director. You may direct a mixed chorus, girl's ensemble, and/or boy's (men's) ensemble.

> *Red Flags:* Are you in the habit of "helping" different sections by singing all the parts (even if the part is out of your natural range)? Are you continually demonstrating vocally? When you conduct, do you use proper upper torso/sternum position or is

your chest collapsed and are your shoulders hunched forward? When you cue sections, what is your head/neck position? Are you elevating and protruding your head and neck? When you cue sections, are you leaning forward and lifting your body weight up? Just as in a previous scenario, the question of how you sit at the piano is a key issue. (You may be in luck and have an accompanist other than yourself!).

Problem Solvers: Singing out of your natural range will cause you to create compensations of your head/neck alignment, tongue, and larynx position. You can help alleviate these problems by using different methods to teach parts. You might choose to (1) use students to demonstrate, (2) play the part on the piano, or (3) have a couple of the musicians with good ears demonstrate while you play the piano. In order to monitor conducting posture, practice conducting and cuing your music in front of a mirror. Also write postural reminders for yourself such as "upper torso/sternum" on index cards and place them in strategic places. Another note about demonstrating: if you sing along with a section you are actually hearing yourself and not the section or the choir! In regard to placement of the rehearsal piano, if you accompany your own ensemble, the same issues apply as in the above scenario.[2]

Choreography

Scenario 2. You are a middle school or high school choir director who directs a show choir and/or a jazz choir.

Red Flags: Where do you rehearse? Are there mirrors? If not, then many students will feel perfectly comfortable vehemently disagreeing with you when you point out specific corrections of choreography. You will then most likely overemphasize positions and talk in a more determined, demanding, and authoritative voice. What is your head/neck position and are your abdominal muscles tightened while you are trying to convince the students of their errors? Is there a microphone for you to use in rehearsal? If not, do you talk over the students talking, over the tape accompaniment, or the live band? Are you looking up at your students on a stage? What is your head/neck position? What kind of vocal projection are you using? What is your energy level? Are you using a healthy "systems balance" of airflow (breath flow/support), phonation, and resonance? Do you create your own choreography? If not, does the person creating the choreography understand the voice and the importance of body alignment and healthy voice use?

Problem Solvers: (1) Get a microphone to use in rehearsals, (2) have students practice choreography in front of mirrors, (3) teach the music thoroughly before putting the music and choreography together, and (4) do not talk or give instruction above other sounds. If you do not create your own choreography, then it is important that the choreographer understand body position in relation to healthy voice use.[2]

Level: College

At the college level there can be a wide range of vocal ensembles ranging from oratorio choruses, chamber choirs, jazz choirs, show choirs, madrigal ensembles, and new music ensembles. Most likely some of the mass choirs will be required for music majors whereas many of the other ensembles will require an audition. The demands and expectations of these groups are usually very high. Also some of these ensembles may require excellent dance skills or actual blocking such as for a madrigals feast.

A *Caution to Conductors*: Ensemble directors must be very careful to place singers in their correct vocal categories. The director might need another alto, but beware, do not slot someone into a section because they can reach all of the notes such as a soprano singing second alto because she can read music well and can reach all of the notes. Do not set yourself up for frustration. This will happen if you have students singing outside their natural tessitura because they will have vocal problems that usually manifest themselves at the most crucial point in the semester, namely, performance time!

Instrumental Directing/Conducting

You may wonder why this has been inserted at this point as mainly we have been examining professionals in the vocal music world. Many School of Music programs certify students as K to 8 general music teachers even if they are instrumental majors. What does this mean? That these students are certified not only to teach a Middle/Jr. High band but also to teach K to 8 classroom general music. There is a problem with this. The curriculum design for an instrumental major often does not include any voice instruction. Even if it does include voice instruction it is often only one semester of class voice. When someone is an instrumental major their instrument is their principal area of private study whereas piano is most often the secondary area of study. Even if an instrumental major is able to move immediately toward the chosen field of band directing, there are inherent vocal pitfalls to watch for as outlined in the scenarios below.

Level: Middle School/Junior High School/ High School

Concert Band

Scenario. You are the director of a band where you have brand new first-time players together with students that have been playing their instruments for at least two years.

Red Flags: Do you raise your voice while giving instructions over misbehaving students? Do you give instructions over instruments playing? Do you sing the melodic line of the instruments over the playing to try to help different sections? Do you give the same level of music to all students? This will most likely cause discipline problems. If the music level meets the newer players then the more experienced players will become bored. On the other hand, if the music level meets the experienced players the newer players will give up. Both of these scenarios are ripe for discipline problems.

Problem Solvers: At the beginning of the year set the rehearsal ground rules. One way to stop a rehearsal is to tap the stand with your baton and give a cutoff cue. If you make the consequences that you establish very clear at the beginning of the year (and carry them out), the problem of straining your voice for discipline over noise will be limited. If you wish to help some students with a melodic line, it is much more efficient to give a cutoff cue and either sing the melody in question or play it on a piano without the background sound causing a decibel level increase to sing over. In regard to music level you will do yourself a great service if you rewrite parts. The way you approach this will depend on the mix of student experience.

Marching Band

Scenario. You are the director of a marching band that is changing from high stepping to Drum & Bugle Corps style marching.

Red Flags: During field rehearsals do you yell instructions without a megaphone? Are you trying to be jack-of-all trades not only by rehearsing the music in concert and field formations but are you also writing the music and marching charts? Are you trying to rehearse the drum line sectionals even though you are not a percussion specialist?

Problem Solvers: If there has never been a band camp before it is especially imperative that a marching band camp be organized for the students to attend prior to the school year starting. It will also be smart to create a parent/volunteer marching band booster club and hire sectional instructors. It is also worth the money and stress reduction to pay someone to write the marching band music charts as well as field charts. It is further worthwhile to hire a drill instructor and percussion ensemble instructor. It is important to remember that the drum line is critical in corps style competition as well as the color guard. Don't try to be a hero and do everything. You will burn out very quickly in body, voice, and spirit (not to mention that you will have a hard time competing with the highest level schools). The high level schools have a separate staff in addition to the director and assistant director for the marching band including: (1) percussion arranger, (2) percussion caption head, (3) visual caption head, (4) color guard coordinator, (5) drill design, and (6) wind arrangement.[3] It is critical for vocal survival to have a megaphone for outside rehearsals. You will also want to appoint an equipment manager and crew to be in charge of a portable sound system for field rehearsals and band camp.

Finale

Teaching Methodology: Commands Versus Tools

One final word that needs to be given here is to encourage each music educator, whether in the classroom, choral rehearsal, band rehearsal, or private lesson, to discern the difference between giving a command versus giving useful tools in regard to teaching anything that has to do with technique. Common commands include (1) sit up straight, (2) breathe deeply, and (3) drop your jaw.[4] The first two commands pertain to both vocal and instrumental music education whereas the third command pertains to vocal/choral music education.

One major postural issue is that of telling students to "sit up straight." When you say that what do you mean? How do you demonstrate this? What word cues do you give? Most often what you demonstrate and tell them in words is interpreted by them as overextending the upper torso/sternum and arching the lower back as discussed in Chapter 1.[4] Remember there may be a difference between learned behavior and what actually is natural alignment. To see the variations, review Chapter 1, Figures 1–11A through 1–11C.

The second common command is "breathe deeply." Isn't it true that if the students knew how to do this then they would have done it already? They need to be taught how to achieve a deep full breath. It is not by working harder that you will achieve this but by learning how to release and open the torso more to allow for a deeper, fuller breath.[4] Review the discussion of respiration in Chapter 1, Figures 1–12A through 1–15.

This third command, drop your jaw, is frequently used by choral directors and voice teachers alike. This is often demonstrated by opening the front of the mouth as wide as possible. It is even further illustrated by asking for a two or three finger-width mouth opening. Exercise extreme caution if you use this because it may actually tighten and not release the jaw joint of the student depending on his/her natural mouth opening. The issue is really about space and the question is: Where does one need to create space? Remember the old song "The knee bone connected to the shin bone . . . ?" Consider the fact that everything is interconnected. What we want to achieve is an efficient resonance tube. Keep in mind that the supraglottic vocal tract begins just above the vocal folds and ends at the lips. Acoustically, the quality of the sound can be affected by how the resonance tube is shaped. We can change the shape by the position of the tongue, soft palate, lips, jaw, and vertical position of the larynx. Other issues include hypo and hypernasality. Therefore, if the question is how to create an efficient resonance tube, then we must consider the interconnectedness of our anatomy. We will not be able to achieve an efficient resonance tube by opening the mouth wide in the front without releasing space between the upper and lower molars. When the mouth is opened in this way, the jaw joint will actually be tightened and the larynx will be held in a higher position.[2] Try an experiment. Gently clench your molars together. Now release the clench and allow space to occur between your upper and lower molars. See how much molar space you can healthily achieve. Notice that when you do this, the mouth opens but it will open as a result of the need to open to allow more space between the molars. Some people like to think of saying "duh." Note that there is no need to press with the chin or the back of the jaw. This is simply one exercise to help create an efficient resonance tube in regard to jaw position. I would highly recommend doing this experiment with your students.[4]

Other common commands include "bring the sound farther forward," "sing into the mask," "project your voice." The quality of the sound is in large part based on the resonance tube. Remember that we have many variables that can shape the resonance tube. Also, the tongue position greatly affects the directionality of the air. If the tongue if too far back then the air will basically get trapped and the singer will have to use more air pressure and muscular tension to push the sound out. The frontal feeling of sound or the projection/placement of sound is an end result. We need to be careful when we talk about "placement" because this makes it sound like the voice is an object that we must push forward. Remember that the shape of the resonance tube and the tongue placement will, in effect, guide the airflow to the end result that we want if we are using our resonance tube and tongue in the most efficient manner.[4]

Caveat: Essay on Personal Musicianship

Personal musicianship skills are as important to the music teacher as they are to the performer. As an elementary music teacher, I have become acutely aware of the unique type of musicianship required of a teacher. As a musician, I am required to sing songs on pitch with and without accompaniment. As a teacher, I must sing songs on pitch . . . even if there are one or two children singing off pitch at full volume.

As a musician, I am required to perform songs at a steady and appropriate tempo. As a teacher, I am required to perform songs at a steady and appropriate tempo . . . even if I am distracted by the rip of Velcro tennis shoes being continually attached and reattached to the carpet.

As a musician, I am required to sing and accompany simple songs from memory. As a teacher, I am required to sing and accompany simple songs from memory . . . even though I am standing rather than sitting at the piano, focusing my attention on the boy in the third row attempting to play the recorder with his nose.

As a musician, I am required to remain focused and expressive for my musical performances. As a teacher, I am required to remain focused and expressive for my musical performances . . . even though I have already been singing for three and one-half hours without a restroom break.

The musicianship required of a teacher is not identical to that of a concert soloist, but it is still musicianship and it must be strong enough to survive the distractions of the classroom.[5]

Brenda Wheat, Music Educator

Acknowledgments. The author thanks Texas Sings! for republication of material from several journal articles.

References

1. Radionoff SL. What music educators wish they had learned. *The Voice Foundation Newsletter*. 1998;October:1–2, 7.
2. Radionoff SL. Warning: teaching can be hazardous to your vocal health! *Texas Sings!* 1997;Spring:19–20.
3. Plymouth-Canton Marching Band. Retrieved July 12, 2007 from http://en.wikipedia.org/wiki/Plymouth-Canton_Marching_Band.
4. Radionoff SL. Commands vs. tools. *Texas Sings!* 2003;Fall:4–5.
5. Wheat B. Personal communication, June 1, 2003.

Chapter 6

Choral Conductors/Participators

$\mathcal{T}$he choral tradition exists in a variety of settings. Outside of school, choral music exists in religious and community settings. In the religious setting there is a wide range of music style and service music. There is music for the traditional service, the contemporary service, and the blended service. A variety of service style and service music is to be found in Catholic, Protestant, and nondenominational churches alike.[1]

Religious Setting

Sanctuary Design

In the religious setting there are different types of sanctuary design and rehearsal room setups. The platforms of four types of sanctuary design discussed here are (1) split sides, (2) center with riser steps, (3) flat floor, and (4) arena style.

Split Side

In the split side platform design seen in Figure 6-1, there are built in riser levels with pews for the choir members to sit in. The organ and piano are often on the same side (stage right). Acoustically it is very helpful in this type of sanctuary design if the rehearsal room is set up with split sides as well. Notice in Figure 6-2 that the rehearsal room is set up with split sides. Even though the piano is in a different position and the conductor is in a position different from that he most often uses in the sanctuary, the choral participants are still able to

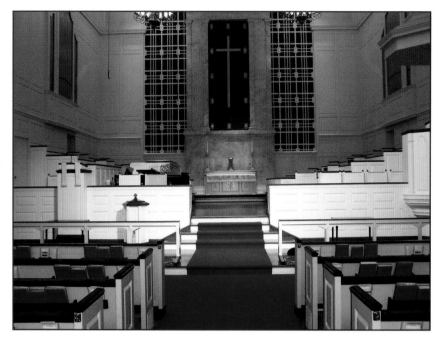

Figure 6-1. Sanctuary of St. Luke's United Methodist Church, Houston, Texas.

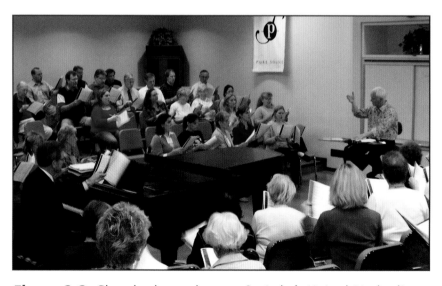

Figure 6-2. Choral rehearsal room, St. Luke's United Methodist Church, Sid Davis, Director of Music conducting with Rob Landes at the piano.

experience similar acoustics. This is especially important for blending and cuing purposes when singing what is considered high church and more traditional music. In this case the primary purpose of amplification is to enhance the natural full sound of traditional service music. This is usually done via hanging microphones which will be balanced for room-appropriateness.

Center

In the platform seen in Figure 6–3, there are riser steps with movable chairs. This allows for versatility of platform use. Note that the organ is off to the side (stage left) and that the piano is on the opposite side. This sanctuary setup lends itself well to different types of music and amplification configurations for contemporary as well as traditional styles of music. The configurations may range from a small trio including drums, bass, and guitar to a chamber orchestra with full choir. It is important in this sanctuary setting that the sound reinforcement

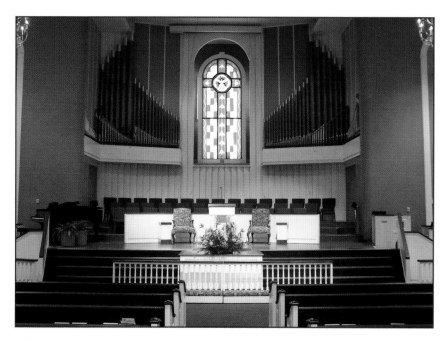

Figure 6–3. Sanctuary of West University Baptist Church, Houston, Texas.

volume and volume distribution fall in line with the following question: How close is the audience to the source? When there are monitors, the sound is louder in the first four rows due to the first few rows hearing sound from both the house system and the monitors.[2] Note in Figure 6-4 that the rehearsal room setup mimics the sanctuary with a center position. Again, this is very beneficial for acoustic and cuing factors for the director and for the choir members as well. It is also advantageous for the choir and director to have the accompanist for that morning's service attend the warm-up time in the rehearsal room prior to the service.

Flat Floor

In the platform setting below (Figure 6-5) notice that the floor is flat and that there is space for a moveable chair setup. In Figure 6-6 the organ has been moved to the side for a different service configuration.

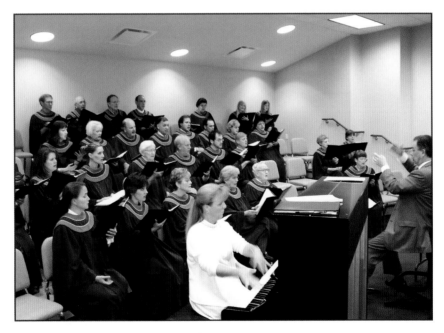

Figure 6-4. Choral rehearsal room, West University Baptist Church, Lee Poquette, Minister of Music conducting with Jan Whitehead at the piano.

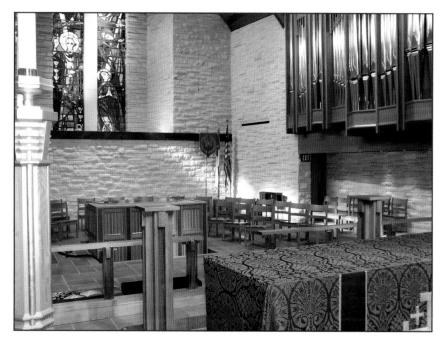

Figure 6-5. Sanctuary of St. John the Divine Episcopal Church, choir setup, Houston, Texas.

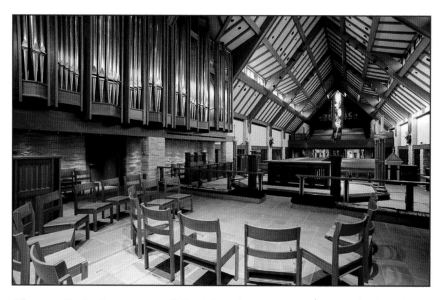

Figure 6-6. Sanctuary of St. John the Divine Episcopal Church, choir setup, Houston, Texas.

The console, as seen below, is movable which permits maximum visibility of conductors and communication with performance groups. In Figure 6–7 all the chancel furnishings were removed to permit a 93-member orchestra with organ and soloists. This was the first major concert after an extensive 18-month renovation that included installation of a 144-rank Letourneau pipe organ from Canada. Every effort was made to improve acoustics, sight line and visibility for maximum clarity of speech and sound. Follow-up measures indicate only a 3 dB loss throughout the room. This was a major improvement from a 38 dB

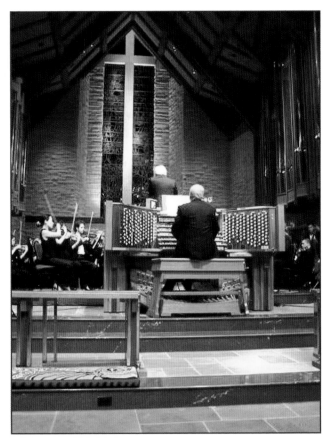

Figure 6–7. Sanctuary of St. John the Divine Episcopal Church, Concert setup, Houston, Texas (UH Concert with Organ and Soloist).

loss from front to back and a 12 dB loss across the chancel prior to the renovation. This renovation facilitates many different types of service configurations as well as concerts and recordings. In fact, it is now the home of the River Oaks Chamber Orchestra (ROCO, Figure 6-8) and many local choral and orchestral groups vie for use of the space as well.[3] The acoustics of this church lend themselves to English choir anthems and antiphonal singing.

Arena Style

In the sanctuary setting in Figure 6-9, notice the size of the space. This arena church seats 16,000 people. In transforming this former basketball venue into a house of worship, the rearrangement of "center court" and the use of sound, lighting, and color (blues and lavenders) were meticulously planned by the architect to help the viewer focus on the center stage and make the space appear smaller.[4] The music for all of the services is amplified. On the platform during

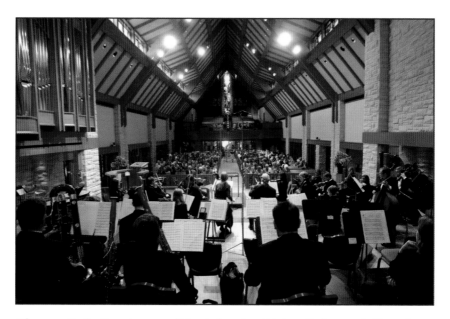

Figure 6-8. Sanctuary of St. John the Divine Episcopal Church, Concert setup (River Oaks Chamber Orchestra/ROCO) Houston, Texas. (Photo by DABphoto)

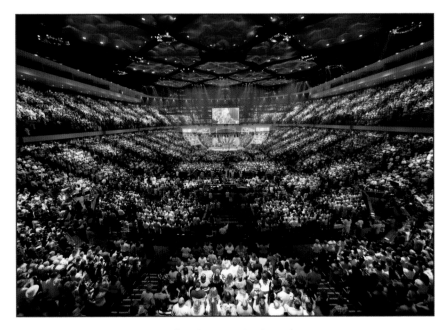

Figure 6–9. Sanctuary of Lakewood Church, Houston, Texas.

services there are four main worship leaders and six ensemble members. There are also 12 ensemble members interspersed among the choir members on microphone per each side of 111 singers.[5] The issue of the rehearsal space setup in this case is significantly different from the other scenarios. There is less need for acoustic similarity between the sanctuary and rehearsal space but a need for good acoustics for blending and hearing oneself and one's section leaders sing. In Figure 6-10, notice the director on an elevated stage. Behind the director are (1) a keyboardist, (2) a drummer, (3) a guitarist, and (4) a male and female leader helping with parts. Also, notice the size of the space necessary for the choir rehearsal.

Style/Service Music

Although there seem to be two main categories of service types which may be defined as traditional and contemporary there are also services that are called "blended" services. These service types can be found in denominational as well as nondenominational churches

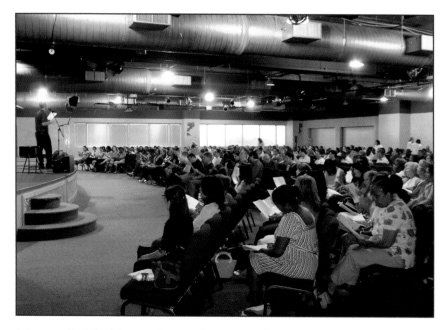

Figure 6-10. Choir rehearsal room, Lakewood Church, Michael Mellett, Choir Director.

alike. These service structures also have different types of service music. Before discussing service music it is necessary to say a word or two about service structures. Some denominations have what would be termed an "order of service" (e.g., Baptist churches), and other churches have what would be called a "structured liturgy for the church year" (e.g., Episcopal churches). Both traditional and contemporary services may be found at denominational churches. There are even denominational churches that call themselves "coffee house" churches. Both traditional and contemporary service structures may be found in nondenominational churches such as bible churches. However, many nondenominational churches tend to lean toward contemporary structures (e.g. Vineyard Fellowship).

Traditional

The terms "traditional" and "contemporary" have variations in definition. In the traditional structure, the service has elements of (1) "familiarity," (2) structure based on denomination, (3) a formulated order of the church calendar, and (4) "presented" music. Typically "presented music" means that there is an anthem by the choir that leads the listener into worship. It is most likely expected that there will be piano and organ music included in the service along with the choral music. In fact, students who study at Concordia College (Lutheran based) all take organ lessons even if they are voice majors. The service structure of the traditional service varies based on the denomination. There will be music to fit the order of the church calendar whether the service has an "order of service" or a structured liturgy for the church year.[2]

Contemporary

Within the contemporary service a wide diversity of style and definition exists. Some consider anything other than high-church music contemporary whereas others consider only current music contemporary. Two churches that have brought contemporary music to the forefront are the Brooklyn Tabernacle and Houston's Lakewood Church (choir roster of approximately 650 members). Cindy Cruse Ratcliff, Lakewood's Music Director, defines their style of contemporary music as "diverse and eclectic. It ranges from Rock to Pop to Rhythm and Blues (R & B) to Gospel and even Latin."[5] She notes that the music often changes style within a song. A song may start as Pop oriented while the bridge is in a Gospel or R & B style. A good example of mixed style would be "Gloria" from Lakewood's CD *We Speak to Nations* which has a Latin Salsa feel but also incorporates a traditional "Gloria" from the Carol "Angels We Have Heard on High."[1]

In the contemporary tradition, amplification is used for singers as well as for instrumentalists. There are many popular brands of sound equipment available such as "Shure" which have excellent wireless microphones available and "Audio-Technica" which is a popular brand of hand-held microphone. The goal is to enhance the sound in the most natural way and that it is "room appropriate."[2] The amount of sound energy created by all of this amplification can trick the singer into feeling like he/she needs to sing louder to be heard. This happens more when there are no monitors for the singers but can happen even with monitors (ear buds as well as wedge style). Many singers who use ear buds actually prefer to use only one to hear room sound and feel the audience energy. Also, when singers try to create the contemporary sound they frequently do this by using tension to stop vibrato (i.e., straight tone) and sound more "pop" in style.

To sing without vibrato actually takes more airflow, not less. This same issue of inefficient production can be found in churches that ask sopranos to produce a young boylike sound to emulate the English Cathedral Choir sound.

Blended

A blended service is one where there are contemporary cultural influences and popular music in a traditional setting.[2] Robert Webber, noted author of many books on worship, prefers to define it as:

> . . . A true convergence of worship rooted in biblical sources, which draws from the great traditions of the church so that it is truly catholic, Reformed, evangelical, and charismatic. It is also deeply committed to contemporary relevance. It is therefore eclectic and engages people in a relationship with God through all forms of music and the arts, including contemporary choruses, drama, storytelling, common gestures, creative movements, participatory involvement, pageantry, and environmental art (p. 1).

It is further interesting to note that according to a recent study by "YOUR CHURCH," blended worship services are on the upswing and the growth of contemporary music in worship has slowed.[6]

Praise and Worship Music

Praise and Worship music may be found in both traditional and contemporary services. Praise and Worship music is defined as a relational or participatory worship experience of adoration. It is a personal expression of worship which is different from the "presented music" of a choir which leads the congregation into worship as discussed above.[2] Some song titles that are used during a time of praise and worship include: (1) We Bring the Sacrifice of Praise, (2) Lord I lift Your Name on High, (3) I Am a Friend of God, (4) Show Me Your Glory, (5) O How I Love Jesus, and (6) There's Just Something About That Name.

The instrumentation for this can take a variety of different forms and may range from acoustic with a single guitar to electric with a full-blown praise band.[2] Figure 6-11 is an example of a praise band with a keyboardist, drummer, percussionist, bassist, guitarist, trumpeter, saxophonist, lead singer, and backup singers. This format does not include a choir.

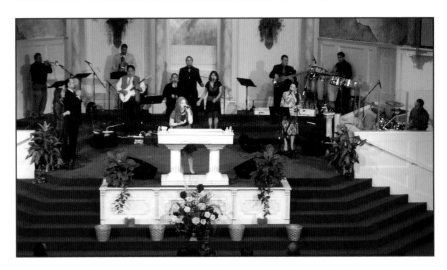

Figure 6-11. Sanctuary of the House of Refuge Christian Church, Pasadena, Texas with the praise band/singers, MelinaAnn Gonzalez, Music Director.

Another example of a praise and worship experience is found in Figure 6-12. This size of this space will have a unique set of acoustical challenges. The challenges will be for tightness of band with choir, band with worship leaders, and band and choir with worship leaders as they direct the congregation toward worship. This will be due to the time delay effect in the arena setting which is much greater than most sanctuaries. Notice that there are elevated steps with split side seating for the choir. Each side has the capacity for 111 choir members totaling 222 for each service. There is a hydraulic lift platform/orchestra pit for the band and there are four worship leaders on stage.[5]

A Cappella

There is one denomination that has a unique history and necessitates mention. The Church of Christ has the distinction of having an a cappella tradition with no instruments in the sanctuary. The Church of Christ was first known as "the Disciples of Christ" and their mission was one of a restoration movement. They wanted to bring the denominations together and what they all agreed on was singing. They base

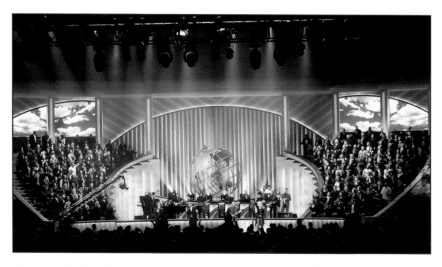

Figure 6-12. Sanctuary of Lakewood Church, Houston, Texas with the praise band/worship leaders/choir, Cindy Cruise Ratcliff, Music Director.

the reasoning of their a cappella tradition on two scripture references: Ephesians 5:19 which says: "as you sing psalms and hymns and spiritual songs among yourselves, singing making melody to the Lord in your hearts"[7] and Colossians 3:16 which says: "Let the word of Christ dwell in you richly; teach and admonish one another in all wisdom; and with gratitude in your hearts sing psalms, hymns, and spiritual songs to God."[7,8] The song leader directs the congregation as "all" sing. In essence, the congregation acts as the choir (Figure 6-13).

Scenarios

Directors: Overview

There are different expectations and job descriptions for the church choir director. Much will depend on the denomination/nondenomination issue as well as the size of the church. In some churches one director does it all: (1) Adult choir director, (2) Youth choir director, (3) Children's choir director, (4) lead Sunday hymns and/or worship

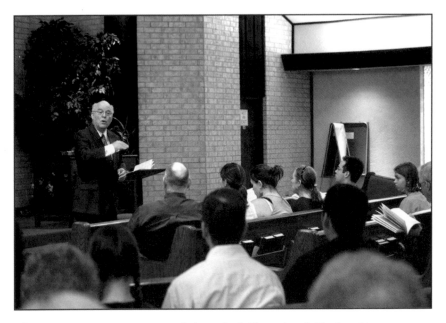

Figure 6-13. Sanctuary of the Alief Church of Christ, Houston, Texas, John Kilgore, Preacher/Song leader/Singing school instructor.

music, (5) play and sing specials, (6) direct handbells, (7) put together special programs, and (8) put together recordings. Factors that need to be considered for directors include (1) rehearsal schedule, (2) performance schedule, and (3) number of ensembles involved in as a participator or director. The volunteer nature of these ensembles and whether or not there are paid section leaders has its own set of pitfalls. In the scenarios below, many of the same things hold true that were mentioned in the traditional choral section of Chapter 5.

Directors: Traditional

Scenario 1. You are the choir director/organist of a volunteer church choir (and there may or may not be paid section leaders). You direct with an upright piano positioned in front of your choir (you accompany all your own rehearsals). You either sit on a regular piano bench or stand.

Red Flags: Where do you rehearse? Are the acoustics good? Do you tend to often play the accompaniment while the choir is singing/learning the music? Do you vocally demonstrate often? How do you structure the rehearsal? How long is the rehearsal?

Problem Solvers: It would be beneficial for you as the director as well as good for the ears of the choir members to work parts a cappella. Other techniques to teach parts that will save your voice would be (1) to play the individual parts on the piano or (2) have section leaders conduct sectionals. It can often feel frustrating if you direct a volunteer choir, when sometimes it seems like they've never before seen a piece of music when you rehearsed it just last week. If you have section leaders one hopes this particular problem will not be quite so bad. Also, careful structuring of rehearsal time can alleviate frustration. Remember that rehearsals are usually at the end of the day. Many choir members have had a long day full of stress and frustration. Because the body is the voice, it is a good idea to do some warm-up exercises for airflow and stress release before working on sound. Also, before working on a choral blend, remember to do exercises that will help each member balance airflow, phonation, and resonance. During warm-up time you can also use difficult rhythms or melodies as vocalizes. If you introduce these new patterns in the warm-up time then they will seem like "old friends" when the choir encounters these rhythms or melodic patterns in the music.

Scenario 2. You are the choir director of a volunteer church choir. You have the luxury of having an accompanist that attends rehearsals.

Red Flags: Are you in the habit of "helping" different sections by singing all the parts (even if the part is out of your natural range)? Are you continually demonstrating vocally? When you conduct, do you use proper upper torso/sternum position or is your chest collapsed and are your shoulders hunched forward? When you cue sections, what is your head/neck position? Do you elevate and protrude your head and neck? When you cue sections, do you lean forward and lift your body weight up? How do you structure the rehearsal? How long is the rehearsal?

Problem Solvers: Singing out of your natural range will cause you to create compensations of your head/neck alignment, tongue, and larynx position. You can help alleviate these problems by using different methods to teach parts. You might choose to (1) use section leaders to demonstrate, (2) have the accompanist play the part on the piano, or (3) have a couple of the musicians with good ears demonstrate while you play the piano. In order to monitor conducting posture practice conducting and cueing your music in front of a mirror. Also write postural reminders for yourself such as "upper torso/sternum" on index cards and place them in strategic places. Another note about demonstrating: if you sing along with a section you actually hear yourself and not the section or the choir!

Directors: Contemporary

Scenario. You are a leader/member of a praise and worship team.

Red Flags: Where do you rehearse? Do you rehearse with a sound system? If not, do you talk (1) over the worship team talking, (2) over the tape accompaniment, or (3) over the live band? What is your head/neck position? Are your arms reaching out and up to the sky? What kind of vocal projection are you using? What is your energy level? Are you using a healthy "systems balance" of airflow (breath flow/support), phonation, and resonance? Are you in the habit of "helping" different sections by singing all the parts (even if the part is out of your natural range)? Are you continually demonstrating vocally? Do you play guitar, keyboard, or piano while you sing?

Problem Solvers: You may rehearse in the actual worship space or in a different space all together. Regardless of the space, it is necessary to rehearse with a sound system if you perform with one. It is okay to raise your arms in worship but you must keep the alignment of the head/neck in its neutral position. Otherwise, you will lose ease and freedom of creating sound. A head/neck position that is elevated and protruded often accompanies the arm position. Look up with your eyes! Be careful to protect your own voice. Do not sing parts that are out of your natural range and do not continually vocally demonstrate. Singing out of your natural range will cause you to create compensations of your head/neck alignment, tongue, and larynx position. You can help alleviate these problems by using different methods to teach parts. You might choose to (1) use worship team members to demonstrate, (2) play the part on the piano, or (3) have a couple of the musicians with good ears demonstrate while you play the piano. You might also consider making a practice tape/CD of parts. Do not talk or give instruction above other sounds. If you sing while you play a keyboard or guitar, the head/neck position is often protruded and elevated in order to "reach" the microphone. Be sure to use either a boom stand or a head set microphone. This will allow for a neutral head/neck position.

Participants

Participants who sing in church choirs range from student and professional musicians to volunteers that may or may not have vocal training or any previous experience. Furthermore, there is often a wide disparity of musicianship and music reading skills. Some participants may be able to sight read music whereas others are able to notice that the black spots on the page go up and down to change pitches. There are also singers and choirs that learn music strictly by rote (imitation) and have no music to read in rehearsal but use text sheets or chord charts.

There are also positions for singers as church choir section leaders available which can be either volunteer or paid positions. The role of the section leader is to be an example for healthy technique and be musically prepared for each rehearsal. Other responsibilities of the section leader may include calling section participants in regard to attendance and also to be a vocal, spiritual, and life encourager. Pacing of body energy is another important issue. Singers have a habit of overextending themselves. Before leaving for choir rehearsal, look into a mirror, raise your right hand and repeat, "I am only responsible . . . for myself . . . and I am not the rescuer . . . of the entire section." Do not forget that your body is your voice. There will be physical ramifications that will affect the voice if a singer does not take time to care for the body. Don't forget to take a water bottle with you to rehearsal.

Scenario 1. You are a member of a church choir.

Red Flags: Do you feel fatigue or tightness in your throat/voice by the end of the rehearsal? Do you notice that your speaking voice is higher by the end of the rehearsal? Do you find that high notes seem difficult for you to sing? Do you have trouble hearing yourself? Do you have visual difficulty reading the music? Do you feel like you have inadequate sight reading skills? Do you feel intimidated like you don't measure up to other singers? Do you feel intimidated when the director is right in front of you while you are singing?

Problem Solvers: If you feel fatigue or tightness in your throat by the end of the rehearsal you have most likely either overused your voice or have been singing with technical inefficiency. If your speaking voice is higher by the end of the rehearsal you have most likely been singing with too much pressure for volume or "reaching" high notes. If you have trouble hearing yourself, it is beneficial to hold your music folder up to use as an acoustic shell to bounce your sound back to yourself. If your choir does not use music folders, it will benefit you to take a folder to rehearsal to use for that same purpose. If it is difficult to visually read the music, ask the director if it is possible to have a CD of the music and/or your part to practice with. This will also help alleviate the pressure to have quick sight reading skills. In regard to measuring up to other singers please remember that there is always going to be someone better than you and there is always someone worse than you. It will be much healthier to expend your energy on 'where am I today and where do I want to be tomorrow.' It truly is wasted energy to focus on other singers. Use your energy in a positive way for self-improvement.

Scenario 2. You are a section leader of a church choir.

Red Flags: Do you find yourself over singing in an effort to "help" those that are singing your same part but incorrectly? Do you find yourself vocally fatigued by the end of a rehearsal?

Problem Solvers: Most often when you sing louder you are actually not helping. Usually a domino effect occurs and everyone simply sings whatever they are singing louder! This can lead to frustration and pushing the voice with pressure which can lead to vocal fatigue. It would be much healthier and better for all concerned if the section leader practiced healthy vocal technique. Some singers say that it is beneficial to think of being in a voice lesson or giving one. It would also be beneficial to hold sectional rehearsals with your section to help teach parts. Furthermore, the placement of where you sit is important. It will be more acoustically beneficial if you sit behind a group of your section instead of in the front row because the sound will travel forward toward their ears.

Community Outreach

In the community setting there are chorales, symphony choruses (often 250+ members) as well as Barbershop, Sweet Adelines, and Madrigal groups. The larger choral works may include such diversity as "The Dream of Gerontius" by Edward Elgar to the well-known work the "Messiah" by Handel. In these large ensembles and in ensembles with orchestral accompaniment it can be difficult to hear oneself sing: Consequently, it is easy to "push" voice production to create more volume in order to hear oneself.

Scenario 1. You are a member of a community chorus and you sing large choral works with an orchestral accompaniment. You have one or perhaps two rehearsals with the orchestra prior to the performance (Figure 6–14).

Red Flags: Do you have difficulty hearing yourself with the addition of the orchestra at the dress rehearsal and performance and therefore oversing? After your first time to sing in this setting do you feel any vocal pain or strain?

Problem Solvers: If you have oversung and you feel vocal pain or strain, you will most likely feel the need to go into "protect mode" where you will hold back energy and air for fear of hurting yourself more. The problem is that by holding back air and body energy you actually make the problem worse. By keeping the energy back in the throat there is more pressure on the larynx. It will be important to let yourself blow airflow on /f/ into your hand and feel that it is not the moving airflow and energy that will hurt you. Remember that sound 'rides' on

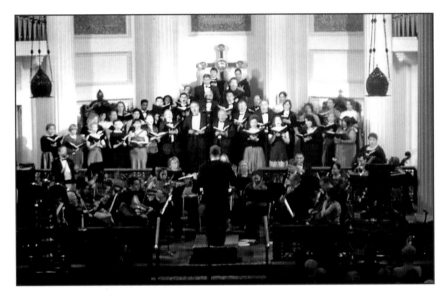

Figure 6-14. Thomas Jefferson University Choir and Orchestra, Robert Thayer Sataloff, M.D. D.M.A, Conductor.

air and the direction that the sound travels is the direction that the air travels. After blowing the airflow on /f/ into your hand, continue with descending slides on /fu- fu-fu/ using a lot of easy breath at the teeth for the /f/ and freedom of sound (IPA vowels).

The Barbershop Harmony Society of America states that it has been in existence since the late 1930s and will soon in fact celebrate its 70th birthday.[9] The stated vision of the society is that it, along with other a cappella organizations worldwide, "is committed to enriching lives in every generation and community through the lifelong benefits of a cappella harmony singing." There are conventions, festivals, and educational conferences which incorporate contests, activities, and training sessions.[10] The sound of the Barbershop/Sweet Adeline style is often described as a "laserlike" pinpoint sound. It is easy to get caught in a trap of using excessive pressure to create a frontal, laser-like sound if one is not careful. Terminology used in this style of singing includes (1) swipes, (2) woodshedding, (3) the "tag," and (4) the "oh yeah." Swipes is defined as changing a chord without breaking the sound, woodshedding in Barbershop refers to making up harmony on the spot (which had occurred in the "woodshed"), and the tag refers to the last sentence of a song. Many of the barbershop songs are written with verse-chorus. Often people do not recognize the verse but say "oh yeah" when the chorus comes in.[11] When you sing barbershop, you must be careful in defining or interpreting commands that are given by the director/leader. When directives are given in a subjective way, unless you've been given the tools to carry out the command and know how to do "it" in a healthy way, you may overwork in ways such as using too much pressure for volume or using excessive glottals for "Punching" the ending chord, and so forth.

Scenario 2. You sing in a "Barbershop Chorus" and are also a member of a Barbershop Quartet (Figure 6–15). Your quartet uses songs

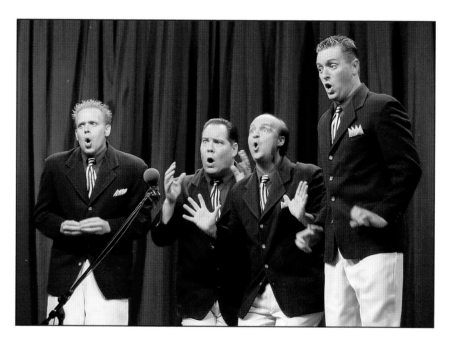

Figure 6–15. Metropolis Barbershop Quartet, James Sabina—Tenor, Brian Philbin—Bass, Bob Hartley—Lead, Mike McGee—Baritone.

as a vehicle for the basis of visual comedy and there is a high degree of movement.

> *Red Flags:* Do you find yourself holding back air or tightening at the throat to have straight tone? Do you do the same thing to "control" the pitch? When working a new song, do you find yourself tightening at the throat when putting together choreography with singing? Do you have difficulty with woodshedding? When you articulate text do you find yourself overworking for clarity of diction?

> *Problem Solvers:* It actually takes more air, not less, to produce a healthy straight tone. Pitch is not controlled by squeezing at the larynx. Pitch is controlled by the ear-brain-systems balance approach as discussed in Chapter 1. When we squeeze at the throat we are generally satisfying a psychological need to "feel" something so that we feel like we are in control. What we are actually doing is feeling a buildup of pressure and glottal tension which can lead to vocal problems. Remind yourself that singing is like golf (technique and follow-through) and not power lifting.

It may be necessary to modify some of the originally intended choreography or you may need to simply practice each element of it with airflow and efficiency of movement until the movement does not interrupt the freedom of airflow and sound production. It is always important to run a fully choreographed routine until every movement and vocal approach becomes second nature. This is necessary to be able to apply the greatest amount of mental energy specifically to the performance of the whole piece. Otherwise, you may be distracted by such thoughts as "How am I going to sing this note while I'm doing this with my leg?" You may need to start the movement slowly in rehearsal and gradually speed it up to tempo until you have achieved a seamless product.[12]

If you have difficulty with woodshedding it will be helpful to learn structures of chords and how they work instead of trying to fly by the seat of your pants. In regard to articulation, clarity is about accuracy not necessarily more of whatever you are doing. If what you are doing is sloppy or inefficient, then doing "more" will simply be more of sloppy or inefficient.

Professional Choirs

Scenario. You sing in a professional choir that performs different music in different performance venues each concert. You sing songs in different styles as well as different languages. Most of the members have a "day job" along with singing in the choir. The choir has an average of 25 performers (Figure 6–16).

> *Red Flags:* Do you notice that you have some vocal tension or fatigue after a rehearsal of reading new music? Do you feel that some of your language skills are inadequate? Do you feel fatigued after your day job?

> *Problem Solvers:* In order to sing in this type of group, it will be imperative that you have excellent sight reading skills and are able to learn new music quickly. It is critical to get past the

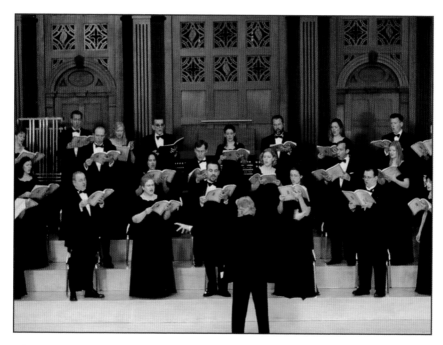

Figure 6–16. Houston Chamber Choir, Robert Simpson, Director. (Photo by Jeff Grass)

basics of the music to get to the real "making" of musical interpretation and nuance. If you feel vocal tension or fatigue after a
rehearsal of reading new music it may be due to difficulties with
your sight reading skills or it may be due to language skills. If it
is due to music reading skills then it will be necessary to spend
enough time in self-preparation to be confident of your part to
be ready for the next group rehearsal. If you are singing a song
in a new language, ask if it would be permissible to record
the rehearsal of that song, and/or find a source to record the
correct pronunciation of the song text for you to practice with.
Because this group performs in different venues, it will be
crucial to be able to form a cohesive sound and adjust to the
new surrounding very quickly. Therefore, knowing your music
intimately is very important. If you have a tendency to feel
fatigued after your day job, it may be necessary to rearrange
your schedule so that you can have some time to eat and rest
prior to your rehearsal if possible.

Conclusion

There are many options available for the singer interested in participat-
ing in choral music. These options exist in a wide array of variations
including: (1) place—school, religious, community; (2) level—volunteer to professional; (3) style—classical, commercial; (4) size—number
of singers from small group to a very large group; and (5) expectation
—time investment/special programs, contests, touring. The objective
is for the singer to find the right fit for him- or herself in regard to the
variations listed above. It may take sampling an assortment of different groups before finding just the right fit. No matter what alternative
is chosen, the basic goals of a singer remain unchanged: holding to the
tenants of general body heath, and vocal health and understanding
the nuance of style and physicality of the options chosen.

Acknowledgments. The author thanks Plural Publishing for republication of materials from the chapter "Artistic Vocal Styles and Technique."
The author thanks all the Churches/Choir Directors/Music Directors/
Ministers of Music, and others who were willing participants in this
chapter. Thank you for your kind attention to detail and cooperation.

References

1. Radionoff SL. Artistic vocal styles and technique. In: Benninger MS, Murray T, eds. *The Performer's Voice*. San Diego, Calif: Plural Publishing Inc; 2006:54-59.
2. Poquette L. Personal communication, July 31, 2007.
3. Gearhart J. Personal communication, August 3, 2007.
4. *Megahouse of Worship/For Lakewood, it's a whole new arena*. Retrieved July 20, 2007 from http://www.chron.com/CDA/archives/archive.mpl?id=2005_3885354.
5. Ratcliff CC. Personal communication, October 15, 2005.
6. *Lighting & Video: Building Blocks of Blended Worship—Church Buyers Guide*. Retrieved August 12, 2007 from http://www.christianitytoday.com/ye/2000/001/5.34.html.
7. *The Holy Bible, New Revised Standard Version*. Iowa Falls, Ia: World Bible Publishers, Inc; 1989.
8. Kilgore J. Personal communication, July 17, 2007.
9. *Welcome to the Heritage Hall Museum*. Retrieved August 9, 2007 from http://www.barbershop.org/web/groups/public/documents/pages/pub_id_062163.hcsp.
10. *Vision and Mission of the Barbershop Harmony Society*. Retrieved August 9, 2007 from http://www.barbershop.org/web/groups/public/documents/pages/pub_id_057333.hcsp.
11. Turnbull S. Personal communication, August 13, 2007.
12. Philbin B. Personal communication, August 19, 2007.

Chapter 7

Performers

There are many different performance genres and venues available to performers. In regard to different genres, the study and performance of style may be discussed in terms of two main broad categories that span a wide spectrum of genres: Classical music and Commercial music. "Classical" is a term which represents many genres including opera, oratorio, art song, symphony, chamber music, and the manner of performance associated with those genres. "Commercial" can include the styles jazz, rock, country, pop, rhythm and blues, big band and swing, alternative, contemporary Christian (CCM), gospel, rap, hip-hop, and heavy metal, to name but a few. These commonly used terms that describe the two main broad categories are recognizable throughout the musical world.[1] That being said, there is one genre not yet mentioned that uniquely stands alone: Musical Theatre. In a recent study conducted by Radionoff, Satterfield, and Lee, it was noted that musical theatre courses are most often not included in the curriculums of commercial music programs of study. Of the 408 programs surveyed (nationally and internationally), only three degree programs in the study had a musical theatre course.[2]

It is interesting to note that Belmont University in Nashville, Tennessee, which has had a commercial degree since the late 1970s, began a separate musical theatre degree in 1997. The rationale for this decision was based on the fact that the commercial music degree did not have any acting or dance elements which are crucial for preparation in the field of musical theatre. This musical theatre degree plan actually has 25 credit hours in theatre and 11 credit hours in dance.[2,3] Therefore, Musical Theatre is listed as a separate performance genre/venue.

The specific performance venues that this chapter covers include the classical genres/venues of opera, operetta, and concert performance, the commercial venues of clubs and large stage venues, and the musical theatre and theatre venues. Other performances of note include CD release parties and private parties. In the following sections are common scenarios that performers often encounter. These scenarios may be familiar to the performer from either personal experience or recognition. Each scenario has corresponding sections entitled "red flags" and "problem solvers." The problem-solvers sections may either help resolve existing vocal problems, or avert potential problems.

Performance Genres: Classical Music

Stage Performance: Opera

Many singers study opera at a university or conservatory and then work in an apprentice program as the next step often performing "opera outreach." In an outreach program singers are customarily hired for 3- to 9-month periods. The contract typically has supporting roles on the main stage (2–3 productions per season) and in the meantime, the singers travel to schools performing operatic versions of fairy tales. Singers routinely perform 2 shows a day, 5 days a week. Often the 45-minute operas begin as early as 8 AM (that is performance time!). Before that, the singer has to wake up, warm up, travel to the school, unload/set up the set, get into costume, and be ready to go by 8 AM to sing. Usually performances are held in gymnasiums/cafeterias that are transformed into performance spaces. Acoustically, this setting is not always friendly. Also, in the warm months, imagine the amount of sweat rolling off you when heavily costumed running around with no air conditioning. After one production the performers would have a short break and then repeat the performance, or they would load up, travel to school number 2, and do it again that afternoon. This type of schedule can make or break a singer and truly show the reliability of one's vocal technique.[4]

Scenario 1. You are performing in Seymour Barab's *Little Red Riding Hood* as the "Wolf." You portray and sing four different voices/characters within the 45-minute show. Along with the wolf, you are disguised as grandmother, little red (offstage), and the woodsman (who comes in at the end of the opera). Your full costume as the wolf has many layers and the choreography for the production is very physical and high energy (Figure 7–1).

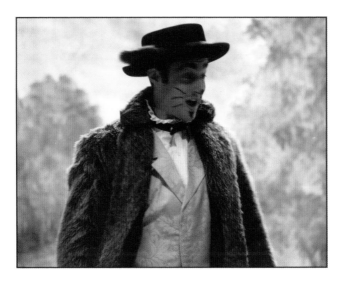

Figure 7–1. Corey Trahan as "Wolf" in Seymour Barab's *Little Red Riding Hood.*

Red Flags: Do you find yourself sweating a lot during setup and during the show? Do you find yourself physically fatigued by the end of the first few days of performance? Do you find yourself vocally fatigued by the end of a performance or by the end of the week?

Problem Solvers: It is immensely important to counterbalance the sweating with enough hydration. It will be critical to pay attention to what your body tells you it needs. Be sure to get enough sleep so that you are ready to wake up early and prepare for every performance. If you are vocally fatigued by the end of a performance, check to be sure that you are not pushing past the vocal boundaries of pitch and use of airflow/pressure for achieving healthy character voices. This is especially important because you are doing four very different voices. If you find yourself physically fatigued by the end of a week-long run it will be important to give yourself vocal/body rest on your day off. Close your lips!

Professional opera singers are often fortunate in that many opera companies have a schedule of alternating two operas such that there is time for voice rest between performances. Things that must be taken into consideration in this livelihood are the number of perform-ances, the number of rehearsals, and the role being performed, travel demands, hotel arrangements, and other factors. When a performer develops the character of his/her particular role, he or she must be careful to preserve the integrity of his/her personal vocal system. By this I mean that the posture and the interpretation of the character "created" by the singer for the role must not interfere with the bal-ance of a healthy technique yet must be convincing in character. When directors and performers begin to develop a character, care should be taken to be sure that the concepts for blocking, costume, and special effects fit within the physicality of the individual.[5] Also, professional opera singers are often in high demand as lecturers and master class specialists.

Scenario 2. You have a dual role in career life. You are a leading international professional opera singer as well as a full-time professor of music at a major university. You have a full studio of voice students, but you are also in demand as a lecturer and master class specialist (nationally and internationally) and you have many professional record-ings and awards under your belt (Figure 7–2).

> *Red Flags:* Do you find that you are somewhat dehydrated after flying to a performance? Are you susceptible to climate changes and differences in allergens? Do you find that you tend to be vocally fatigued on certain days? Are you teaching a full+ load of singers in your studio along with lecture classes?

> *Problem Solvers:* It will be beneficial to start hyperhydrating two to three days prior to flying. Often there is not much down time between flying into a venue and then performing. Therefore, it will be necessary to arrive well hydrated in order for the vocal folds to vibrate properly. Be sure to pack the recommended "Travel Pack" for yourself that is outlined in Chapter 3. Things like saline spray and Nasalcrom (over-the-counter allergy buffer) may be very beneficial. Also Entertainer's Secret and Throat Coat tea can help soothe a feeling of dryness and can help thick mucus to dissipate. It will be beneficial to arrange your teaching load such that you are not overtaxing the voice prior to leaving for a singing engagement. This also holds true for a singing engagement at the university where you teach or a performance near where you live.[6]

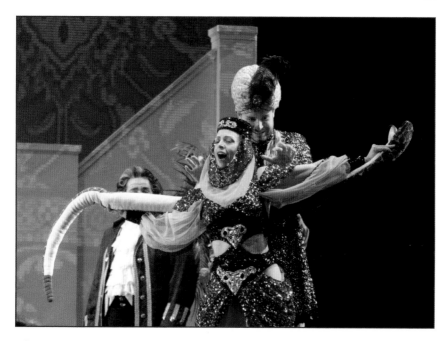

Figure 7–2. Katherine Ciesinski as "Samira" in John Corigliano's *The Ghost of Versailles*, Moores Opera Center. (Photo by Pin Lim/ Forest Photography)

Stage Performance: Operetta

The term "Operetta" began as a small-scale operatic work but developed by the middle of the 1800s into a distinct genre. A well-known English form of operetta comes from Gilbert and Sullivan—Sullivan's musical style set to Gilbert's social satire. The two scenarios below demonstrate scenes from the *Pirates of Penzance*.[7]

Scenario 1. You are singing a role that demands wielding a sword and dueling while singing (Figure 7–3).

Red Flags: Do you feel off balance with the sword and forward movement? Do you feel that your body weight is primarily on the balls of your feet? Is your stomach pulled in and tight due to self-consciousness of your costume? Do you ever find yourself gasping for breath near the end of the song after dueling?

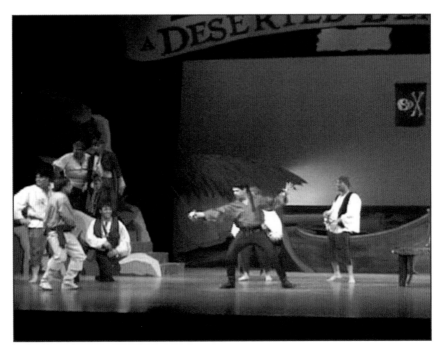

Figure 7-3. John Gremillion as the "Pirate King" in a rehearsal of *Pirates of Penzance* (singing while dueling).

Problem Solvers: It is imperative that you practice with the sword during rehearsals to become comfortable with the weight of the sword and how this affects the freedom of your body movement. It is also important that you practice the choreography for the duel while doing the airflow exercises discussed in Chapter 2. This is a perfect example of a "multi-tasking" exercise described there. It is also necessary to practice either in costume or something similar to allow yourself to feel comfortable and breathe normally even if you do notice that your stomach seems to pooch out more than you'd like. Be sure to practice the movement in a mirror to monitor efficient position as discussed in Chapter 1. Usually, if you find yourself gasping for breath by the end of the song it is not just a problem of breath at the end of the song—it has actually progressively been getting less and less efficient. Remember that mirrors don't lie. Practice the song with and without the choreography in front of a mirror to monitor body position as well as the release of the abdomen.

Scenario 2. You are vocally tired, overloaded vocally (too much voice use during the day), and have to sing a difficult role during technical rehearsal week without the aid of any amplification (although there will be amplification during performances).

> *Red Flags:* Do you feel fatigue, hoarseness, or strain at the end of a rehearsal? Do you feel like you have to push or shove to get the high notes to come out? Do you notice that you are thinking that you have to "fill the hall" with sound and find yourself forcing to do this? Do you notice that your mid/high range is difficult to sing? Are your high notes flat? Is your vibrato rate slower than usual? It is very common for the high range to be difficult, the high notes to be flat, and the vibrato rate to slow down if you are pressurizing the sound and forcing it with tension at the neck or glottis (space between the vocal folds).
>
> *Problem Solvers:* One of the best ways singers can be kind to their vocal folds is by efficient vocal production during rehearsal time. If you are tired vocally or if there is no amplification during practice then marking is a very smart technique to use in rehearsal. Healthy marking is achieved by using good breath support and singing easily at a comfortable dynamic level. The singer may also choose to take the extreme high notes down an octave. Marking does not mean singing softly with inadequate breath support.[8]

In addition, cool-downs are an important part of the routine at the end of long performances or rehearsals. The important issue is to reduce the fatigue and pressure at the larynx and to increase the ease of phonation. If the voice is somewhat tight or fatigued, descending vocal slides, lip trills, or lip bubbles with a lot of breath and support using medium, easy dynamics may be used until your voice feels that it is settled and in its comfortable register (Figure 7–4).

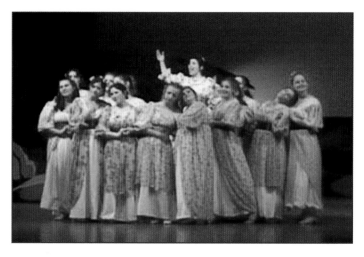

Figure 7–4. Kitty Karn as "Mabel" marking the high "C" during a rehearsal of *Pirates of Penzance*.

Concert Performance: Stage

Repertoire for a classical solo concert may be quite varied. Years ago, the typical classical solo concert performance was comprised of an evening of "Art Songs." This has changed over the years in that many classical singers now also perform what are considered standards from musical theatre as well. It is often easier for an operatic singer to sing from "legit" or classically based musical theatre repertoire (i.e., *Oklahoma, Carousel, Phantom of the Opera*) rather than from other styles of shows such as *Rent* or *Jesus Christ Superstar* unless he or she has had training in understanding what makes the integrity of a certain style and how to implement those stylistic tools for an appropriate sound quality.[9]

Scenario. You are performing in a recital at the Madrid Theatre in Los Angeles. The recital features a program that is varied to showcase your versatility (Figure 7–5).

> *Red Flags:* As you are preparing for this recital do you find that your tessitura gradually gets higher after singing for an extended

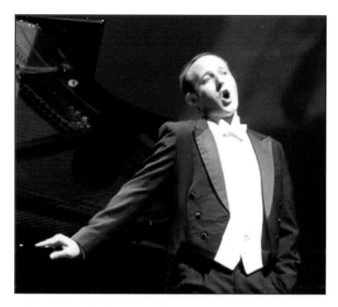

Figure 7–5. Corey Trahan in concert at the Madrid Theatre in Los Angeles.

period of time? Does this make a difference in how you program the recital for the most efficient use of the voice? Do you find that it makes a difference in technique if you sing arias and art songs or musical theatre and pop songs first?

Problem Solvers: In rehearsal, it would be beneficial to journal how the voice responds when you change the order of the song program. If you notice that your tessitura seems to gradually get higher after singing for an extended period of time then you will want to organize your recital program so that the lower tessitura songs are at the beginning and the higher tessitura songs are at the end. Also, if you notice that your voice seems to respond in a more grounded way technically when you start the program with classical songs first, then be sure to do so! You always want to pay attention to what your voice and body tell you. It may be mentally how you approach different styles which cause a certain physical activity to occur—nevertheless —it is what it is. Listen to your body.[4]

Concert Performance: Intimate Setting

Scenario. You are singing in a very intimate setting. There is close proximity between the singer/pianist and performers/audience members (Figure 7–6).

> *Red Flags:* When you first sing in an intimate setting do you find that you are taking shallower breaths than normal? Does it feel awkward to make eye contact with your audience—especially the front row? Are you used to having to "fill the hall" in performance? Are you in the habit of overdoing articulation from other venues of performance?
>
> *Problem Solvers:* It would be highly beneficial when you begin booking performances in intimate settings that you prepare for the experience by singing in a similar setting prior to the event. This is not only an overall space issue but also regards your comfort level with people in very close proximity while singing. This awkwardness will especially hold true for the first few performances of this type. If you feel self-conscious you may pull your body in physically. This will affect the power

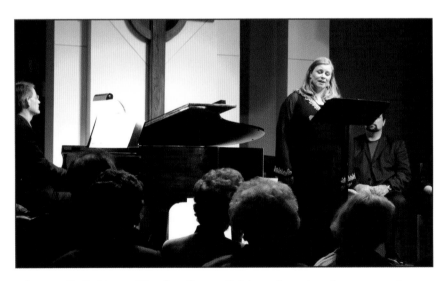

Figure 7–6. Tracy Rhodus Satterfield performing in an evening of Schubert Art Songs (Liederabend) with Col Canto.

source (managed airflow) which, in turn, will impede sound and musicality. Also, because this is an intimate setting you will want to be sure to visually make eye contact with many in the room so that no area or grouping feels left out. In this setting you are free from the burden of "superhuman" projection—no need to think "fill the hall." When performing in this type of venue think "small screen" versus "large screen" or TV versus theatre. What works on a big stage can be distracting or seem affected to the audience in a more intimate setting. There can be different options such as using whisper and other colorations in this setting.[10]

Performance Genres: Commercial Music

Singers who perform in clubs, give concerts such as CD release parties, and sing for private parties and galas have a number of issues to deal with. They are often expected to sing in a smoky environment with little air circulation for three or four 45-minute sets a night with 15- to 20-minute breaks between sets. The only place that they can go to get away between sets may be either the bathroom or their own car! They often fight bad sound equipment or frustrating sound engineering problems, sing, play an instrument, and even dance as well as do their own booking which means "voice on" during the day for booking and performing (often without much rehearsing) during the evening.

The different variables that the professional singer often has to deal with include: (1) the number of concerts, (2) type of environment—noisy, smoky, dry, dusty, crowded, (3) dialogue between numbers, (4) talking between sets to audience/promoters, (5) where to go between sets, (6) accompaniment—live band and so forth, (7) choreography, (8) sound equipment, (9) sound engineer, (10) warm-ups, (11) rehearsal time, and (12) promotion and booking.

Clubs

Scenario 1. You are the lead singer of a band but also sing backup on a few songs. The style is a mix of folk, swingy/bluesy/jazz, bluegrass, Cajun, and South American traditions (with a bit of rock/country).

There are core members that play rhythm/lead guitar, drums, and bass. Other live performance instruments may include fiddle, mandolin, banjo, and percussion instruments (Figure 7–7).

> *Red Flags:* Do you rehearse with a full band but no sound system? Do you perform without putting a cage around the drums? Do you take a band sound system or use the house system when you perform at clubs? Do you use the house sound engineer or one of your own? What is the size of your rehearsal space? Does it resemble any of the clubs where you perform? Are there trustworthy ears in the house when you run a sound check for balance?

> *Problem Solvers:* If you rehearse with a full band, it will be to the singer's favor to rehearse with a sound system—otherwise, the singer will overwork and push to acoustically match what the instruments are putting out. Also, if you use the house system at a gig, be sure that you have plenty of time for sound check—especially the first time that you perform at a venue. This is important for the band as well as the sound engineer. Many clubs do not allow outside sound engineers to use house

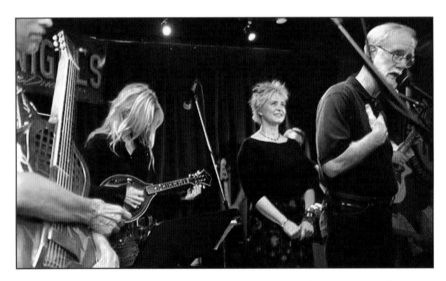

Figure 7–7. Sugar Bayou with lead singer April Rapier, performing at the "Mucky Duck" being introduced by Rick Gardner.

systems. This can prove difficult if the sound engineer does not routinely balance the type of group that you sing in. It would be very beneficial to know and mark out with tape on your rehearsal space what the stage size will be at a new venue. Otherwise you may not be used to a cramped space and feel restricted or the space may be larger than you are used to and you may get winded trying to move and pay attention to all sides of the performance space.

Scenario 2. You are a drummer/lead singer that sings Rhythm and Blues music (Figure 7–8).

Red Flags: Do you notice yourself taking a high chest breath? Do you sit comfortably on your stool or are you leaning forward arching your lower back? Are you under a high stress level? Do you find your high range cutting out by the mid/end of a show? Do you need an extended warm-up time? Do you have to lower the keys of songs that you had previously had an easy time with? Do you book your own shows? Do you use a headset microphone or boom stand? Do you use an inner ear monitor?

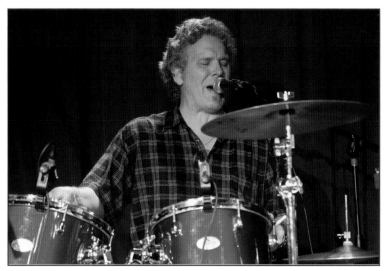

Figure 7–8. Doyle Bramhall, Texas Singer/Songwriter/ Drummer, performing at "House of Blues" Dallas, Texas. (Photo by Kirk R. Tuck)

Problem Solvers: Be sure that you practice with efficient lower back positioning while sitting on your stool. If you practice with an arched back then you will perform with an arched back. Remember that this body alignment will cause problems with being able to get a good, relaxed, deep abdominal/diaphragmatic breath. In the long run, inefficient use of airflow may cause you to overwork at the neck to try to control power of the voice. This, in turn, may start to cut off the upper range and you will lose flexibility of your voice. As a result you may need to lower some song keys. If you book your own shows then you are using not only voicing during shows but a lot of voicing to call/set up, and confirm bookings. It will be vocally beneficial to use a headset microphone or boom stand and/or an inner ear monitor. You will sing with more ease if you can hear yourself!

CD Release Party

Scenario. You are the female vocalist singing with a jazz trio for a CD release party (Figures 7-9 and 7-10).

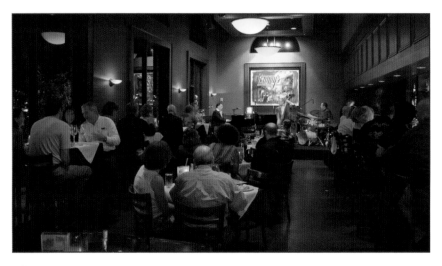

Figure 7-9. Matt Lemmler Trio in a CD release party at Tommy's Seafood Steakhouse. (Photo by Pin Lim/Forest Photography)

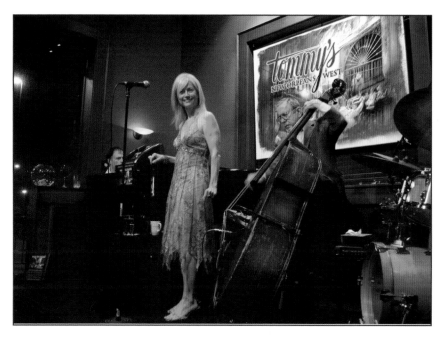

Figure 7–10. Diane Landry, female vocalist with the Matt Lemmler Trio. (Photo by Pin Lim/Forest Photography)

Red Flags: Have you performed in this club prior to the CD release party? Do you routinely sing with this trio? Have you used the sound system before? Is there time to warm up and check sound before the club is full of people? Where do you go during your breaks? Do you talk between sets? Do you have water to drink on stage or near the stage? Is there any smoking in this club?

Problem Solvers: If you have not performed in a given venue prior to a CD release party, it is highly recommended that you arrive early enough to become comfortable in the space. It will also make a difference in your comfort level as a singer if you have performed with the trio prior to this main event. If you have only performed a few times with the trio, it would be to your benefit to be sure to request a little extra time for sound check to allow for enough preparation to go through entrance/ exits of songs and talk about style and tempo.

Gala Event

Scenario. You are a gospel singer and have been asked to be the special feature artist at "An Evening of Inspiration." In your career you sing solo concerts, sing in a duo group, and sing backup for an internationally acclaimed gospel artist. You have recorded a solo CD, a duo CD, and have been a featured artist on church CDs as well. Together, your husband and you pastor a church. You sing specials at your home church as well as other churches. You are a full-time mother of three and you have recently been going through chemotherapy treatments for cancer while still traveling and performing (Figure 7–11).

> *Red Flags:* Do you notice that you are vocally hoarse and physically tired after your cancer treatments? Do you have nausea or loss of appetite after your treatments? Do you observe that you have a difficult time finding the energy to take care of the household at this time?

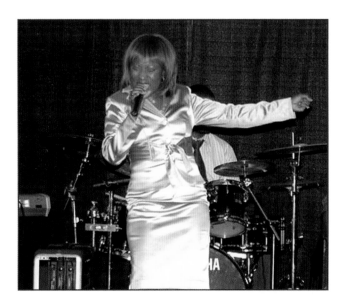

Figure 7–11. Rosalyn Brunswick-McDuffie, gospel singer, at "An Evening of Inspiration" in Beaumont, Texas. (Photo by Alfred Beverly)

Problem Solvers: It is not uncommon to experience some vocal hoarseness and physical tiredness after cancer treatments. The American Cancer Society states that the tiredness factor is not a normal type of tiredness but a "bone-weary" tiredness and that this fatigue is caused by low red blood cell counts.[11,12] It is important to remember that your body is your voice. Therefore, anything that affects your body while you are going through cancer treatments has potential to affect your voice. Remember that chemotherapy is designed to kill cancer cells. The side effects of this treatment may include abdominal pain, nausea, vomiting, and infection. You may also lose your appetite. According to the American Cancer Society, it may be helpful to eat small portions every 2 to 3 hours until you feel better before trying to go to a normal mealtime schedule. They also state that this problem usually decreases over time.[11] It will be important to consult your physician in regard to the recommended time of rest to allow the body to 'recharge' its energy so that you will be able to schedule the time between treatments and performing in order to achieve the most healthy results for physical healing as well as for healthy, safe performing. It is imperative that you enlist help with taking care of your household and children as necessary. In fact, you may wish to enlist family or friends to spend time with your children during and after treatments to allow for recuperation time.[13]

Large Stage Shows

Scenario. You are the lead singer in a Latin Pop band. Your band has been asked to be a featured band at Super Bowl XXXVIII at Reliant Stadium in Houston, Texas (Figures 7-12 and 7-13).

Red Flags: Are you familiar with performing in this type of venue? Are you familiar with the expectations of time for set up, sound check, and time to get on/off the stage? Are you used to the type of sound delay that occurs in this size of arena? Do you usually perform on a stage where the audience is dark and there are spotlights on the stage or are you used to seeing such a large crowd? Do you have inner ear monitors?

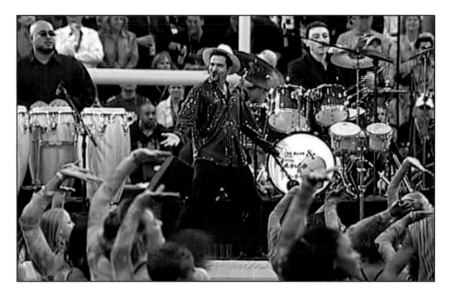

Figure 7–12. "Walter Suhr and Mango Punch!" a Latin Pop Band created by Walter Suhr, performing at Super Bowl XXXVIII at Reliant Stadium, Houston, Texas.

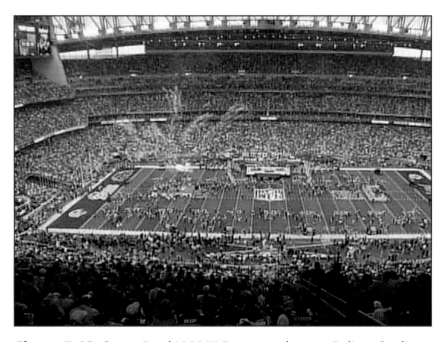

Figure 7–13. Super Bowl XXXVIII Pregame show at Reliant Stadium, Houston, Texas.

Problem Solvers: When singing in a large venue such as a sports stadium, you must be sure that there are no major distractions to what your job is. It would be very easy to get caught up in the energy of the stadium. Be careful to not oversing and to let the microphone do the work. It is your job to entertain and energize the crowd—not to overwork to try to "fill the stadium" with sound—that is the job for the sound engineer. Be sure that you are comfortable with your monitor situation—it will make a big difference in the ease of your performance. Also, be sure that your band and all the people involved understand the tightness of precision necessary to put on a great show—after all, you do want to be asked back! If you are not used to seeing such a large crowd I would suggest that you ask for time prior to the event to be able to stand on the field and become comfortable with the venue.

Performance Genre: Musical Theatre

Introduction

In Musical Theatre, the performance practice "sound du jour" has historically gone through changes. In the book *The Complete Professional Audition* by Cohen and Perilstein, one can find songs and musicals in a variety of categories. Vocally, there is variation in singing style depending on when a musical was written. In the first chapter, Cohen[14] organizes shows into groups that encompass similar styles ranging from Country-Western influence (*Oklahoma*), Teens/Children (*Into the Woods*), Pop/Rock (*Jesus Christ Superstar*), and Outcasts/Underdogs (*Hairspray*) to name a few. In regard to different vocal sounds, there are musicals that are considered more classical in sound such as *Oklahoma* and *Phantom of the Opera*, whereas *Rent* and *Jesus Christ Superstar* use a contemporary pop/rock sound.[9]

Those who perform the principal roles of a musical production are rarely asked to perform or play more than one character in an evening. However, *Jekyll and Hyde*, for example, demands two very different vocal productions from the male lead in every performance. It is very difficult to perform at the extremes of range and style every night and stay healthy. Other shows that require principals to perform more than one character in an evening include: (1) *Into the Woods*, (2) *The Apple Tree*, and (3) *I Love You, You're Perfect, Now Change*. Also, in *Sunday in the Park with George* the cast plays different roles in the first and second act. Other difficulties include the use of character voices such as: (1) Little Bird (*Seussical*) and (2) Adelaide (*Guys and Dolls*). When creating a character voice, one has to be careful not to pass the point of healthy coloration and effect whether it is producing a cartoonlike voice or using nasalance. Each singer has a window of opportunity for coloration and effect and must experiment with how far he or she may go from the central balance point and still have integrity of technique. Another interesting twist is bringing Disney characters to life on the theatrical stage. It can be difficult to create an inanimate object such as a clock, teapot, or candle (*Beauty and the Beast*) and keep integrity of body alignment (potential to adversely affect airflow).[9]

Unfortunately, music theatre is not quite as kind to its singers as the opera world is in regard to rehearsal and performance schedules. Singers are often expected to sing up to 8 shows a week—with 2 and even 3 shows a day including a children's early morning program. Roles like the male lead in *Jekyll and Hyde* with its vocally demanding extremes are difficult enough for 1 show a day let alone 2 or 3. Other difficulties include such things as tap dancing from table to table while singing or singing while doing a back bend where your ankles hold you suspended from a metal bar. Unfortunately, the thing that usually suffers is not the staging and choreography but the voice.[5]

Musical Theatre

Scenario 1. You are performing the role of the "Witch" in Stephen Sondheim's *Into the Woods*. You wear a prosthetic mask in Act 1 and the "ugly" witch is required to walk with a limp and a hunch. The prosthetic mask is gone in Act 2 when you become "beautiful" but you wear a corseted top (Figures 7–14 and 7–15).

> *Red Flags:* Do you find it difficult to sing comfortably wearing the prosthetic face mask that you must wear in Act 1? Is it possible to breathe through your nose at all? Do you find it difficult to take a full breath in the hunched position? Are you holding your ribs and hip stiff when limping? Do you notice that you are using mainly rib/chest breathing in both Act 1

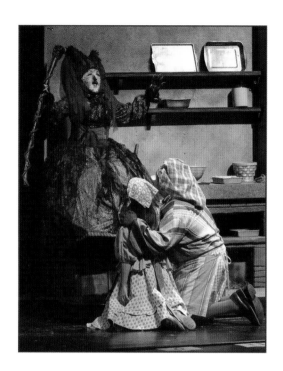

Figure 7–14. Kristina Driskill as the "Witch" in Act 1 of Sondheim's *Into the Woods*. (Photo courtesy of WVU Photographic Services).

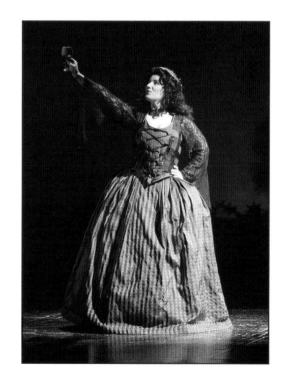

Figure 7–15. Kristina Driskill as the "Witch" in Act 2 of Sondheim's *Into the Woods*. (Photo courtesy of WVU Photographic Services).

due to the body positioning and Act 2 due to the corset? Is it
difficult to sing the same phrase lengths in performance on one
breath that you were able to comfortably sing in rehearsal? Do
you find yourself running out of air too quickly? Do you have
the necessary type of body microphone available?

Problem Solvers: When you go to your costume fitting be
sure to take a full breath as you normally do when singing
and keep your rib cage expanded during the fitting. It is also
highly recommended (if the costume shop will allow) that you
practice with the corset in rehearsal. This will allow you to
become accustomed to the feeling. The same holds true for
other costume issues such as the prosthetic face mask. It could
be a difficult psychological challenge if you are a nose breather
but are unable to do so with the mask on. It also will be
beneficial to practice during technical rehearsal week with the
body microphone in order to become comfortable with it.

Scenario 2.   You are performing the lead role "Laurey" in Rogers and
Hammerstein's classic *Oklahoma*. Normally, in the dream sequence
there is a double who is a ballerina that performs en pointe as Laurie.
Because you are a highly talented ballerina as well as singer, you will
be performing both (Figures 7–16 and 7–17).

Red Flags: Do you find it difficult to get a full breath to sing
the song after you dance? Do you notice that you experience
fatigue by the end of the show? Do you feel that the high notes
are difficult? Are you used to speaking in the accent needed for
the character?

Problem Solvers: It will be imperative to practice going back
and forth from thinking and being in "dance posture" to
"singing alignment." As this musical was not written for one
performer to normally both sing and dance, you will actually
need to practice for the body transition to become quick for it
to be useful and efficient. It also will be beneficial to practice
some of the dance sequence followed by airflow and body
movement for singing using the consonant /s/, /f/, or consonant
combination /sh/ to remind the body of how it needs to respond
for sound production. The next steps would be to (1) practice
long tones on comfortable pitches following some of the dance

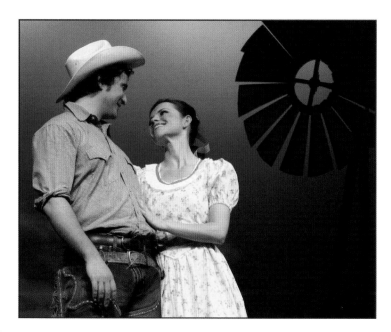

Figure 7-16. Chrisi Carter as "Laurey Williams" in Rogers and Hammerstein's *Oklahoma.* (Photo by Scott Magee)

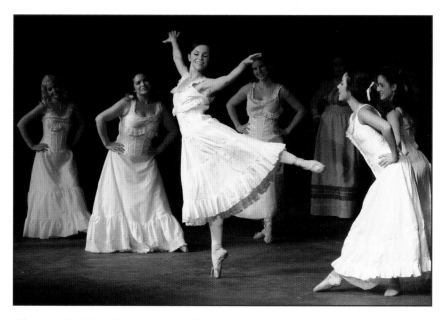

Figure 7-17. Chrisi Carter dancing to "Many a New Day" in *Oklahoma.* (Photo by Rick Nielsen)

sequence, (2) practice melodic patterns from the songs on a comfortable consonant/vowel combination, (3) chant the text of the song on a single pitch, and (4) sing song phrases with text and melody together before singing the entire song following the dance sequence. In regard to the speaking voice, be sure to practice the accent with exercises that will allow for technical efficiency such as chanting the monologues on a single pitch. It is very easy to get into a compensatory behavior for creating an accent. The back wall of the pharynx behind the mouth is often overopened which creates excessive space and inefficiency of resonance.

Performance Genre: Theatre

Many of the same issues apply to the professional actor/singer as to opera and musical theatre performers. In nonmusical theatre the actor may play one role throughout an evening's performance, or he/she may play several different characters. This becomes a problem when the actor has to create believability with such diverseness as being a German doctor, a Spanish grandmother, and a high school cheerleader all in one show. Again, when creating characters such as these, you must give the illusion of the characters without compromising the vocal system and be sure to work within the parameters of your own physicality. In Houston's Alley Theatre production of *The Devil's Disciple* by Bernard Shaw, one actor played both the British General Burgoyne and the commoner Uncle Titus; the comportment and voice of each were vastly different (Figures 7–18 and 7–19). The same actor, in the twohander *Stone's in His Pocket* by Marie Jones, was required to use six different Irish dialects with a character age range from 6 to 78. Indeed, all the characters in this production were portrayed by only two actors. The virtuosity required to satisfy the textural and pitch demands in such instances is very taxing on the voice and can do damage without proper vocal technique.[5,15]

Scenario. You are playing two very distinct roles in a production. In the first Act, you play a very rough, commoner with a physical deformity. In the second Act you play a General in the British Army with very erect posture and absolutely pristine social/physical behaviors and demeanor.

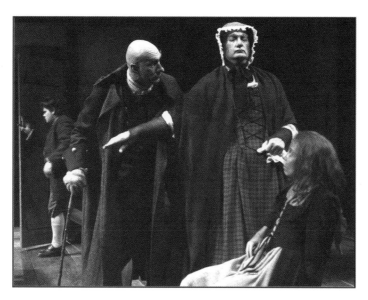

Figure 7-18. Todd Waite in Houston's Alley Theatre Performance of *Devil's Disciple* as Commoner "Uncle Titus" with Paul Hope as "wife of Uncle Titus." (Photo by Jim Caldwell)

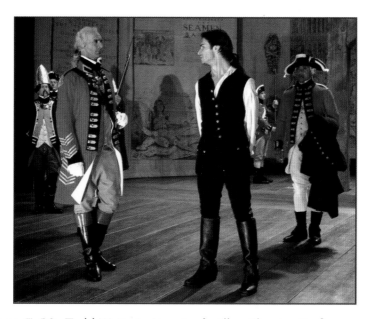

Figure 7-19. Todd Waite in Houston's Alley Theatre Performance of *Devil's Disciple* as "General Burgoyne" with Ty Mayberry as "Dick Dudgeon" and David Rainey as the "sergeant." (Photo by Jim Caldwell)

Red Flags: Do you find that by the end of a week of performances that you feel out of alignment in body? Do you notice any
change in breathing patterns or any holding of breath? Do you
find that you wake up with a feeling of tightness in your neck,
back, or rib cage? Do you notice any tightness in the soft palate?

Problem Solvers: After performances it is necessary to do body
stretching to be sure that the body alignment is centered for
the next night's performance. It would be beneficial to include
head/neck stretches along with rib cage stretches and center
of gravity alignment. Along with body stretching, it will be
necessary to do airflow and sound balancing exercises. This is
important as it is possible to lose the center of the "system's
balance" when performing two such diverse characters.

Conclusion

Currently, career marketability of young singers requires a broader
ability than ever before in regard to genre. One singer who was strug-
gling for years to find his niche in the business was being told
"although you can sing leading male roles, you're too short to be cast
in them" or "you sound too operatic for most of the current Broadway
roles," and so forth. After several discussions with his "team" (i.e.,
voice teacher, coach, stage director/acting teacher) he decided to pur-
sue this career in roles that suited his body type, and personality, and
spanned as many genres that he could successfully perform and stay
true to each genre's demands. The solution was to continue to study
to develop the voice to sing leading roles but auditioning and performing supporting/character roles, both character baritone and character tenor roles. The choice to play "second fiddle" has enabled this
singer to consistently work in opera and musical theatre along with
unlimited opportunities to be the "leading male" in recital series, oratorio and shows that are not physically and vocally discriminate. In
fact, this singer is now booked a year in advance with such diverse
performances as "Seymour" in *Little Shop of Horrors*, "Remendado"
in *Carmen*, "Gastone" in *La Traviata*, and last, performing in a recital
"Hooray for Hollywood," to name a few.[4] It is of note to mention that in
2002, an entire month's issue of *Opera News* (August)[16] was devoted

to the crossover phenomenon between opera and the theatre. There has never been a time when being a crossover singer has been as important as now.[9]

In order to have longevity of career, healthy technique is essential! There are common threads of airflow management, body alignment, and stylistic tools that must be attended to in order to maintain a healthy career. It does not matter if you specialize in classical or commercial music; this holds true across genres and broad categories alike.

Acknowledgments. The author thanks *Journal of Voice* for republication of material from the article "Preparing the singing voice specialist revisited." The author thanks *Texas Sings!* for republication of material from several journal articles. The author thanks Plural Publishing for republication of materials from the chapter "Artistic Vocal Styles and Technique." The author wishes to thank all the performers who were willing participants in this chapter. Kudos to all of you! You are all amazing.

References

1. Radionoff SL, Binkley CK. *Commercial Singing for Classical Singers.* Professional workshop presented at The Voice Foundation's 25th Annual Symposium Care of the Professional Voice; Philadelphia, Pa; June 1996.
2. Radionoff SL, Satterfield TR, Lee E. *Commercial Music: A Survey of Degree Granting Institutions.* Poster presented at the 37th annual Symposium Care of the Professional Voice, Philadelphia, Pa, June, 2007.
3. Halbert M. Personal communication, May 2007.
4. Trahan C. Personal communication, July 2007.
5. Radionoff SL. Preparing the singing voice specialist revisited. *Journal of Voice*; 2004;18,513–521.
6. Ciesinski K. Personal communication, July 2007.
7. Randel DM. *The New Harvard Dictionary of Music.* Cambridge, Mass: Belknap Press of Harvard University Press; 1986.
8. Garrett JD, Radionoff SL, Rodriguez M, Stasney CR. *Vocal Health.* Lynnewood, Wash: Blue Tree Publishing; 2003.
9. Radionoff SL. Artistic vocal styles and technique. In: Benninger MS, Murray T, eds. *The Performer's Voice.* San Diego, Calif: Plural Publishing Inc; 2006: 51–59.
10. Satterfield TR. Personal communication, July 2007.

11. *What Happens After Treatment?* Retrieved August 31, 2007 from http://www.cancer.org/docroot/CRI/content/CRI_2_2_6X_Moving_On_After_Treatment_of_Ovarian_Cancer_33.asp?rnav=cri.

12. *Chemotherapy.* Retrieved August 31, 2007 from http://www.cancer.org/docroot/CRI/content/CRI_2_4_4X_Chemotherapy_33.asp?sitearea.

13. Brunswick-McDuffie R. Personal communication, August 12, 2007.

14. Cohen D, Perilstein M. *The Complete Professional Audition: A Commonsense Guide to Auditioning for Musicals and Plays.* New York, NY: Back Stage Books; 2005.

15. Waite T. Personal communication, September 28, 2005.

16. Rauch RS (ed). *Opera News,* August, 2002.

Index

A

Abdominal muscles, 12
Acoustics
    formant frequencies, 25
    and hertz, 25, 26
    pitch, 25, 26
    singer's formant, 26-27
Alexander technique, 2
    head/neck position, 4
Alignment
    basic stance, 3-8
    and body weight gravity center, 3
    feet, 3
    head/neck position, 4-6
    jaw position, 6-8
    knees, 3-4
    neck/head position, 4-6
    shoulders, 4
    sitting, 8-9
    standing, 3-8
    sternum/upper torso, 4
    upper torso/sternum, 4
Analgesics, 96
Anatomy
    abduction/adduction muscles, 16
    arytenoid cartilages (larynx),
        14-15
    cricoarytenoid muscles, 16-17
    cricoid cartilage (larynx), 14-15
    cricothyroid muscles (CT), 16-17
    extrinsic muscles, 18-19
    intrinsic muscles (larynx), 15-18
    larynx, 13-20
    phonation, 12-20

recurrent laryngeal nerve, 28
respiration, 10-12
sternohyoid muscles, 19
strap muscles, 19
stylohyoid muscles, 19
superior laryngeal nerve, 28
supraglottic vocal tract, 21
thyroarytenoid muscles (TA),
    16-17
thyroid cartilage (larynx), 14-15
torso, 11
vocal folds, 12-13, 20
Antihistamines, 95, 96
Articulation
    consonants,
        class/anatomic area, 31, 32, 33
        fricatives, 32
        glides/liquids, 33
        manner/shaping of sounds, 31,
            32, 33
        nasals, 33
        stops/plosives, 32
    and jaw, 30
    mechanisms, 30-32
    and vocal technique, 45
    vowels, 30
Arts medicine centers, 82-83
Arts medicine/professional voice
        care, 75-76. *See also* Vocal
        pedagogy; Voice science
        history
    diagnoses, functional, 89, 91-92
    general body health, 92-101 (*See
        also main heading* Health,
        general)

213